HEALTH CARE POLICY IN THE UNITED STATES

edited by

JOHN G. BRUHN
PENNSYLVANIA STATE
UNIVERSITY-HARRISBURG

Health Care Policy in the United States

John G. Bruhn, editor

Physician Participation in Medicaid Managed Care
Sunday E. Ubokudom

Healing the Social Body: A Holistic Approach to Public Health Policy
Elizabeth R. Mackenzie

Directing Health Messages toward African Americans: Attitudes toward Health Care and the Mass Media
Judith L. Sylvester

Gender Justice and the Health Care System
Karen L. Baird

Who Cares for Poor People? Physicians, Medicaid, and Marginality
Margaret M. Hynes

Health Care Reform: Policy Innovations at the State Level in the United States
Larry E. Carter

Telemedicine in Hospitals: Issues in Implementation
Sherry Emery

Helping Survivors of Domestic Violence: The Effectiveness of Medical, Mental Health, and Community Services
Judith S. Gordon

Families and Their Health Care after Homelessness: Opportunities for Improving Access
Lisa M. Duchon

FAMILIES AND THEIR HEALTH CARE AFTER HOMELESSNESS

Opportunities for Improving Access

LISA M. DUCHON

Routledge
Taylor & Francis Group
NEW YORK AND LONDON

First published 1998 by Garland Publishing, Inc.

This edition published 2013 by Routledge

Routledge
Taylor & Francis Group
711 Third Avenue
New York, NY 10017

Routledge
Taylor & Francis Group
2 Park Square, Milton Park, Abingdon,
Oxfordshire OX14 4RN

First issued in paperback 2016

Routledge is an imprint of the Taylor and Francis Group, an informa business

Library of Congress Cataloging-in-Publication Data

Duchon, Lisa M.
Families and their health care after homelessness : opportunities for improving access / Lisa M. Duchon.
p. cm. — (Health care policy in the United States)
Revision of the author's thesis (Ph. D.)—New York University, 1997.
Includes bibliographical references and index.
ISBN 0-8153-3146-0 (alk. paper)
1. Family—Medical care—Pennsylvania—Philadelphia—Longitudinal studies—History 20th century. 2. Urban poor—Medical care—Pennsylvania—Philadelphia—Longitudinal studies—History 20th century. 3. Homeless persons—Medical care—Pennsylvania—Philadelphia—Longitudinal studies—History 20th century. 4. Poor—Housing—Health aspects—Pennsylvania—Philadelphia—Longitudinal studies—History 20th century.
I. Title. II. Series: Health care policy in the United States (New York, N.Y.)
RA564.9.H63H38 1998
362.1'086'9420974811—dc21

98-42309

ISBN 13: 978-1-138-96953-7 (pbk)
ISBN 13: 978-0-8153-3146-9 (hbk)

For Dennis

Contents

Tables and Figures

Preface

When I first began my literature review for this research, I was surprised to come across a published dissertation from 1969 titled, "Studies in the use of health services by families on welfare," by a doctoral student at the City University of New York.[1] The research was based on a sample of poor mothers in New York City. The results showed that families on welfare used clinic facilities more than private physicians. In contrast, the general population relied primarily on private physicians for medical care. Almost 30 years later, I find myself in the same position of publishing a dissertation on the use of health care services by welfare families in New York City. For the most part, the findings then still hold today. My research is quite different, however, in looking specifically at the effects of homelessness on the use of primary care services.

In 1969, family homelessness was not the social problem it is today. As noted in a sourcebook on homelessness, "Today poverty increasingly means the risk of losing one's home," with the "marginally housed" facing the on-going risk of becoming the "literally homeless."[2] Women and children are estimated to comprise almost 40 percent of the total homeless population. Yet, homelessness is largely a *temporary* experience for families.[3] This research is unique in examining the utilization of health services of families after most are no longer homeless.

As a student and former practitioner of public administration, I am interested in the role that bureaucracy plays in shaping our understanding of homeless families and families on welfare. Bureaucratic labels are an important means of acquiring access to a variety of services.[4] We would consider all families living in a shelter as "homeless," but not all families that are without their own place to live are residing in a shelter, where they may gain access to referrals for extremely scarce housing. Bureaucratic labels tell us who and how many are eligible for services, but not who or how many are in need of assistance. We know very little about formerly homeless families or their use of health services once they are no longer labeled homeless by the bureaucracy that once sheltered them. The findings from this study begin to address this knowledge gap.

On a more personal note, while conducting this study, I faced my own challenges with affordable housing, and access to health care, based on my bureaucratic label as a university doctoral student. I often found myself in disbelief at the thought of life imitating *research.* It seemed that way when I felt mistreated by the bureaucracy of the university's health clinic, my only source of health care, and every time I had to move—usually out of one illegal sublet into another. I was moving more often than many of the homeless families in our research study. My primary trade-offs for subletting affordable, rent-stablized apartments were living with pests and plumbing problems, and having to leave at the owner's whim. I count my blessings that I have never been without a home in New York City. But my own experiences have given me a deep appreciation for the hundreds of families in our study who experienced homelessness and the disruptions of moving frequently, or struggled to stay in their own place, despite lousy conditions.

My own struggles, I knew all along, were temporary. They only strengthened my resolve to tell the stories in our data. Since finishing my dissertation, I have found stable housing, and now can choose my own physicians through a relatively generous employer health plan. Unfortunately, as the research presented here shows, many poor families continue to face access barriers to health care even after they are no longer homeless.

Yet, by comparing homeless families to poor, housed families, this research also shows their commonality in poverty's grip. Compared to the general population, the mothers in our study, mainly black or of Hispanic descent, have high rates of chronic health problems, low educational attainment, poor employment histories, low marriage rates and long-term dependence on public assistance. Although the gap between rich and poor has widened considerably, these statistics aren't so different from what Pomeroy reported almost 30 years ago.

The health care system, by contrast, has evolved dramatically in that time. Just in the half-dozen years since I began working on this research study, enormous changes have occurred with the rapid growth in Medicaid managed care across the country and an overhaul of the nation's welfare programs. Even the family shelter system in New York City, which previously offered shelter—no questions asked—has policies requiring families to "demonstrate that they have no other housing options available" before they are allowed access to emergency shelter.[5] These policy changes have profound implications for poor families, because they are changing the bureaucratic labels that confer entitlements to health care, housing, and cash assistance.

Unfortunately, no one knows how the interplay of these policies will affect people's lives and well-being over time. My hope is that, over time, we will at least have a health care system that permits coverage for and access to appropriate and high quality health care services based merely on citizenship and need, and not on the status of one's age, income, employment, housing, welfare or enrollment in a university. Universal access to health care will not end poverty nor prevent family homelessness, but it will go along way towards mitigating the unintended consequences of bold reforms that seek to make poor families more responsible for their own health and welfare. Our ability to inform the design of policies that are socially and ethically responsible to poor families, depends, in part, on undertaking research, such as this, that acknowledges the dynamic nature of people's lives in a dynamic policy environment.

NOTES

1. Pomeroy, R. (1969). *Studies in the use of health services by families on welfare*. New York: City University of New York, The Center for the Study of Urban Problems.
2. Fantasia, R., & Isserman, M. (1994). *Homelessness: A sourcebook*. New York: Facts on File, Inc., p. 17.
3. Shinn M., Weitzman B. C., Stojanovic, D., Knickman J.R., Jimenez L., Duchon L., James S., Krantz D. (1998). Predictors of homelessness from shelter request to housing stability among families in New York City. *American Journal of Public Health*, 88 (12), in press.
4. Vedlitz, A., & Alston, J. (1983). Welfare terminations and benefit reductions: What program recipients can tell policy planners. In R. Goldstein &

S. Sachs (Eds.), *Applied Poverty Research* (pp. 138-147). Totowa, NJ: Rowman & Allanheld.

5. Department of Homeless Services. (1998). *Services at the department of homeless services*. New York: City of New York, p.2.

Acknowledgments

As with every book, this one required input from many, not the least of whom were the staff of Garland Publishing who took an interest in my dissertation, upon which this book is based. My sincerest thanks to editor Kristi Long and Dr. John Bruhn, the series editor, for choosing to include my work in this series. My thanks as well to Rebecca Wiplfler for her patience and helpfulness.

Many others helped me intellectually, emotionally and financially towards completing the arduous task of writing a doctoral dissertation. I am indebted to my dissertation advisor, Beth C. Weitzman, for inviting me to work on a longitudinal study of poor housed and homeless families in New York City, funded by a grant from the National Institutes of Mental Health. I am grateful for the intellectual guidance that Beth and Marybeth Shinn, principal investigators of the project, provided me during the four years I worked on this research. My heartfelt thanks also goes to John Billings and Leanna Stiefel for cheerfully serving as members of my dissertation committee, and to Jan Blustein and James Martin for their valuable suggestions.

The information presented represents the collective efforts of many other individuals as well—administrative staff, interviewers, and other graduate and work-study students at New York University—who were dedicated to the research project. In particular, I would like to thank Pei Chen, Larissa Labay and Daniela Stajanovic for their tireless efforts and commitment to the project.

Friends and family also sustained me in many ways. I appreciate my parents, Claude and Helen Duchon, for always believing I could accomplish anything I set my mind to. My sincerest thanks, as well, to Lyn Rice, for creating the figure included in this book, and for being my lifelong friend. And finally, I thank Dennis Andrulis, whose unwavering love, understanding, patience, generosity—along with his fabulous cooking and wine collection—kept my spirits lifted, throughout all the struggles with writing and re-writing.

Regardless of the wonderful support of others, I take full responsibility for the errors or weaknesses that may be found in this work.

Introduction

"All progress tends toward the solution. Someday we will be surprised . . ."

—Victor Hugo, from *Les Miserables,* 1862

Three decades since Medicaid was implemented, a vast literature in the field of health services utilization supports the conclusion that Medicaid has improved access to health care for poor families. Qualifying this assertion is recognition that poor families still under-utilize primary care services compared to their more affluent counterparts, when health status is taken into consideration.[1] They also still use clinic and hospital-based facilities disproportionately compared to the general population.[2] Much less research has examined differences in patterns of utilization *among* poor families, who are no more homogeneous than the "general" population. Thus, improvements in public health care have benefited the poor generally, but necessarily uniformly.

Many factors—call them the new realities of urban living—may play a role in differentiating patterns of health care use among the urban poor. Street violence, domestic violence, substance abuse, AIDS and homelessness have made life for poor, urban families more dangerous and unhealthy than ever. For a variety of reasons that are no doubt complexly intertwined, some poor families have fared better than others against the risks of urban living. Given the diversity of experiences and characteristics of low-income families, we would expect the poor, as a group, to have a variety of health care utilization patterns.

Beginning in the 1980s, homelessness became one of the risk factors for families living in conditions of poverty.[3] By the mid-1980s, the U.S. Conference of Mayors estimated that female-headed families made up one-third of an estimated 2.5 million homeless people in the U.S. Experts studying the phenomenon have blamed the growth in homelessness on structural conditions such as the 1981-82 recession, accompanied by unemployment and changes from a manufacturing-based to a services-based economy; cutbacks in federal housing support and other social programs during the Regean Administration; a reduction in the purchasing power of public benefits; and a shrinkage in the supply of low-cost housing, rising in part, from the "gentrification" of urban neighborhoods.[4–7] Funds for federally subsidized housing programs were cut over 69 percent between 1981 and 1989.[8] The country's largest landlord, the New York City Housing Authority, had a waiting list of approximately 200,000 families by the end of the 1980s.[9] Personal characteristics such as problems with mental illness, alcoholism and drug abuse have also been attributed to the rise in the homelessness of the last decade.[10,11] "Most important," says Burt, "homelessness is associated with poverty and the accompanying inability to afford housing."[12]

The field of homeless research on families emerged during the rapid growth in the number of homeless families in the 1980s. Most studies in this area have looked at families who are residing in a homeless shelter. Indeed, the *operational* definition of family homelessness has largely been a "construction of the shelter system."[13] Research is only beginning to focus on the *dynamics* of family homelessness. An understanding of how the dynamics of homelessness relate to health care utilization can help determine whether experiences from living in shelter explain the differences in health care use that researchers have found in studies that compare sheltered families to housed families.[14] An important question is whether those differences disappear after families are no longer homeless.

If the experiences of homelessness tend to lead to a given pattern of health care use, then what is that pattern after the family is no longer labeled homeless because it is no longer living in a shelter? And what is it about the shelter experience—its duration, mobility between shelters, experiences resulting from shelter, services targeted specifically to people in shelter—that might lead to homeless families using health care differently from other poor families?

It could be that consequences of the shelter experience affect families' connection to the health care system. The consequences could be personal, such as substance abuse problems, family break up, and/or health problems, or more structural in nature, such as policies or institutional practices that lead to the loss of public assistance. Other health care utilization consequences of homelessness could be isolation from private doctors, or relocation from shelter to a place that is unfamiliar, unsafe and/or lacks access to private physicians. All could possibly influence whether a family becomes connected to a private doctor or clinic as a regular source of care, or uses public institutions. The source of care is an important concern for access, given the research findings showing that hospital-based sources of care (outpatient departments and emergency departments) provide less continuity of care.[15]

Perhaps families who become homeless are more likely to have different patterns of health care use than other poor families even before they enter shelter. The conditions of housing instability, from not having one's own place and being doubled up, or from moving frequently among family and friends—which often proceeds "official" homelessness[16]—may make it more difficult, compared to poor families with stable housing, to find a regular source of care, especially with a private provider.

Answers to these questions have important policy implications for any city that provides services to homeless families. For example, if homeless families have relatively weak links to mainstream health care providers after leaving shelter, a fitting response is to help families connect with appropriate providers in their new neighborhoods. If aspects of the shelter experience, such as a long stay or the type of shelter used, are associated with later health care use, policies should focus on improving the delivery of health care services that are targeted to or are indirectly available to homeless families.

Previous studies on homeless families have shown that sheltered mothers are more likely than poor, housed mothers to lack a regular source of care and to use emergency departments and clinics rather than private doctors' offices.[17] Researchers have not examined whether these patterns persist after families are re-housed. Families in New York City's shelter system are, in general, provided health care through affiliations with public hospitals and community clinics.[18] Once families are re-housed, usually after a year,[19] they may have trouble finding a medical home, because they lack a connection with providers in their new neighborhoods.

This book focuses on the health and health care use of families after they have left the shelter system, with the first three chapters dedicated to a review of relevant literature. Chapter 1 begins with an overview of early studies on the relationships between housing and health, concluding with a summary on residential factors that often precipitate family homelessness. Chapter 2 highlights research on homelessness and health, and the connection of each to poverty, followed by a summary on the limitations of cross-sectional research on homeless families. Chapter 3 features literature on the characteristics of homeless families, including comparisons of their health and health care use to poor, housed families and other populations.

The research design, as presented in Chapter 4, include hypotheses that address several aspects of the relationship between homelessness and health care use among poor families. Unique to this research is treating shelter use as one part of a broader concept of "residential instability." The term encompasses mobility before and after homelessness, in addition to shelter use itself. Conceptual models of health care utilization have largely overlooked residential instability as a factor in utilization outcomes. Though "residential mobility"[20] is included as a factor in the widely-used Behavioral Model of Health Services Use, it is rarely incorporated into studies of either general populations or specific groups. The Behavioral model, the conceptual framework for this research, is modified to examine how aspects of residential instability are related to poor families' current patterns of health care use.

The research is based on self-reported data collected during a follow up study of 543 poor New York City mothers who were first interviewed in 1988. All mothers were receiving public assistance at that time. About half entered shelter sometime in 1988 or later, and half never used shelter. Only a handful of homeless mothers (n=11) were still living in shelter approximately 4.5 years later when we re-interviewed them. We also included their children (n=765) in the follow up study.

Chapter 5 compares "ever-sheltered" and "never-sheltered" families on the various characteristics and factors included in the analytical model. The results of multivariate analyses, as discussed in Chapter 6, show that having ever used shelter is very predictive of where families currently seek health care, even after they are no longer homeless. This finding, and many others, along with a discussion of recent developments in state and federal health and welfare policies, provide the backdrop for a discussion, in Chapter 7, of policy options that may help formerly homeless families find an appropriate medical home, and may improve accountability in the delivery of health care for all poor families.

The recommendations reflect a sense that the cycling and re-cycling of families through welfare and emergency shelters may become even more dynamic with the implementation of the federal Personal Responsibility and Work Opportunity Reconciliation Act of 1996, which set time limits and other restrictions on public assistance entitlements. As a new age of welfare reform dawns, and the climate of managed care competition for Medicaid patients has both heated up and begun cooling off, the relationship between residential instability and health care use among poor families will continue to have important policy implications for New York City and other urban communities as well.

NOTES

1. Davis, K., & Rowland, D. (1991). Financing health care for the poor. In E. Ginzberg (Ed.), *Health Services Research*, Cambridge, MA: Harvard University Press, 93-125.
2. Dutton, D. B. (1978). Explaining the low use of health services by the poor: Costs, attitudes, or delivery systems? *American Sociological Review*, 43 (6), 348-368.
3. Fantasia, R., & Isserman, M. (1994). *Homelessness: A sourcebook.* New York: Facts on File, Inc.
4. Ibid.
5. Burt, M. R. (1992). *Over the edge: The growth of homelessness in the 1980s*. New York: Russell Sage Foundation.
6. Jacobs, F. H. (1994). Defining a social problem: the case of family homelessness. *American Behavioral Scientist*, 37 (3), 396-403.
7. Bassuk, E. L. (1991). Homeless families. *Scientific American*, 265 (December), 66-74.
8. Fantasia, R., & Isserman, M. (1994).
9. Ibid.
10. Burt, M. R. (1992).

11. Jacobs, F. H. (1994).

12. Burt, M. R. (1992), p.6.

13. Berlin, G., & McAllister, W. (1994). Homeless family shelters and family homelessness. *American Behavioral Scientist*, 37 (3), p. 423.

14. The Stanford Center for the Study of Families, Children & Youth. (1991). *The nine studies of homeless families, children and youth.* Stanford, CA: Author.

15. Newacheck, P. W., & Butler, L. H. (1983). Patterns of physician use among lowincome, chronically ill persons. *Medical Care*, 21 (10), 981-989.

16. Thrasher, S. P., & Mowbray, C. T. (1995). A strengths perspective: An ethnographic study of homeless women with children. *Health & Social Work*, 20 (5), 93-101.

17. Ibid.

18. Office of Mental Health. (1988). Programs for homeless children and families. *Homelessness performance report*, Albany, NY: Department of Social Services, State of New York.

19. Shinn M., Weitzman B. C., Stojanovic, D., Knickman J.R., Jimenez L., Duchon L., James S., Krantz D. (1998). Predictors of homelessness from shelter request to housing stability among families in New York City. *American Journal of Public Health*, 88 (12), in press.

20. Andersen, R. M., & Newman, J. F. (1973). Societal and individual determinants of medical care utilization in the United States. *The Milbank Memorial Fund Quarterly*, 51(1), p. 107.

Families and Their Health Care after Homelessness

CHAPTER 1

An Overview of Research on the Link between Housing and Health

Before homelessness became a "hot topic" of social science research, for decades, numerous studies were conducted on the effects of residential mobility and housing conditions on health and health care use. Highlighted below are some of the more salient findings and theories as they relate to housing, mobility, health, and health care use.

HOUSING CONDITIONS AND HEALTH

The term poverty, itself, is suggestive of poor housing conditions, which are in turn associated with various health problems.[1] For example, dampness and coldness, which are favorable conditions for molds, have been highly associated with childhood asthma and depression in adults.[2] Other conditions that may affect health include indoor air pollution (e.g., lead, asbestos, formaldehyde), fires and other accidents, pest infestations, noise, lack of privacy and overcrowding. Living density is an important factor in the spread of infectious diseases. Poor housing conditions have been associated with higher rates of miscarriage, stillbirth, infant mortality and birth of a child with congenital abnormalities.[3]

Duvall and Booth, however, highlight the inconsistencies of research findings on the relationship between housing quality and health.[4] A large, comprehensive study in the 1970s, by Wilner and colleagues, compared 400 black families in Baltimore, who were moved from "slum housing" to a new public housing project, with a comparison group of families from the area who were not re-housed.[5,6]

After ten re-interviews of families, only modest differences in health were found. It was impossible to determine which or whether housing conditions were responsible for the decrements in health that were reported.

Nevertheless, that substandard living conditions are common among poor, housed families may help explain the similarities in health problems afflicting homeless and poor, housed families, as described in the next chapter. Even being re-housed from shelter is no guarantee of adequate housing conditions. According to a New York City survey by the Housing Preservation and Development Department, 13 percent of households occupied by "previously homeless" persons were in a unit with five or more "maintenance deficiencies," while only 7 percent of households without previously homeless persons occupied such a unit.[7] "The highest incidence of previous homelessness is associated with public assistance recipients whose crowded conditions are caused by doubling-up in their household."[8]

RESIDENTIAL MOBILITY AND HEALTH

Research regarding the effects of residential mobility on health date back to the 1930s.[9] Earlier research tended to focus on the health consequences of particular kinds of moves, such as those associated with "slum clearances," moving to suburban areas, or into new "satellite" towns.[10] According to Stokol and Schumaker's review of residential mobility and health, research from the 1950s and 1960s identified moving as a "stressful life event."[11] The "stress model" theory stipulates that the experience of moving can "tax or exceed [individuals'] coping abilities and adaptive resources."

Various studies have linked mobility with symptoms such as depression and gastrointestinal problems, which may persist for several months after a move. For the majority of Americans, though, changing residence is voluntary and does not lead to detrimental health problems. The *inability* to move could even be more harmful than relocation. Researchers have found that the adverse effects of moving are mediated by the "predictability of the move," and the "controllability of the new environment."[12] Stokol and Schumaker expand the predictability-controllability characterization of mobility to a broader situational context that includes the "person-environment fit" and the person's "comparative appraisal of previous residential situations."[13] The concepts may very well apply to poor or homeless families, although these findings were based largely on middle class populations.

RESIDENTIAL MOBILITY AND HEALTH CARE USE

Residential mobility was often cited as an important determinant of health care utilization in early studies on the subject.[14] In particular, length of time at a residence influenced whether families had a regular source of care. More recently, Poland, Taylor and Hayes found that for (poor) families living in Grenada, West Indies, those residing in the study area with the longest residential histories had the highest levels of service use.[15]

In a recent U.S. study, 10 percent of children from families who had moved three or more times did not have a regular provider for obtaining sick care, compared to only 3 percent for children who had never moved, and 7 percent for all U.S. children.[16] Emergency room use was also associated with high residential mobility.

PATHWAYS TO HOMELESSNESS

Residential instability, as defined in this study, refers to several gradations of risk for homelessness, including homelessness itself. The first is the high degree of mobility that may result when families are moving from one "doubled-up" situation to another—among family members or friends—because they do not have their own place (even though they are not technically homeless, as defined by the shelter system). Often families turn to the shelter system after wearing out their social networks.[17] The second is living in precarious conditions, such as unaffordable rent or unsafe housing conditions, which may put a family living in its own place at risk of becoming homeless. The third is the experience of living in a homeless shelter, which may include mobility within the shelter system, for example, from a welfare hotel to a Tier II family apartment (see Appendix A). Shelter may also bring a measure of relative stability, however, for families that reside in the shelter system while waiting their turn in the queue for permanent housing. Families may be at risk for more instability after becoming re-housed, depending on the mother's level of independence, the quality of the housing and neighborhood, and other circumstances, which could re-start a cycle of residential instability.

The literature is lacking in research that documents how patterns of health care use may relate to or change with the dynamics of residential instability. The forms of residential instability that can lead to urban family homelessness are varied, such that patterns of health care use might vary with them. A summary of one of the few studies to look at the ways in which families become homeless provides a broader context for understanding the dynamics of family homelessness.

Families in New York City who were interviewed at the time they were requesting shelter were generalized into three categories of pathways to homelessness.[18] For about 43 percent of the families studied, homelessness came about from a disruption in an otherwise relatively stable situation. Eviction and rent problems were the most common sources of instability. Building problems, such as rodents and lack of heat or water, physical abuse or the threat of it, and other interpersonal problems in the household also led to a loss of housing.

Another 44 percent of families requesting shelter in New York City were mostly young, small families who had never had their own place to live. In the last year before entering shelter, nearly all had been doubled-up with their parents, other relatives, or friends, and left because of problems with the primary tenants. Most entered shelter within one month of leaving their doubled-up arrangement. These families fit an image of the "multigenerational welfare family," with few resources beyond public assistance.[19]

A minority of homeless families (13%) experienced a "slow slide from primary tenancy to homelessness."[20] Once living in stable housing, one-third had left their place within the past year. Another third had not lived in their own place for one to two years, and another third had not for more than two years. This group averaged the highest rate of mobility in the past three years (3.2 moves). They also lived in more crowded conditions and were more likely to have had experiences with substance abuse, mental hospitalization, and child protection services, compared to other homeless families.

With this background in mind, the next chapter presents literature on the aspects of health and health care use associated with homelessness.

NOTES

1. Freund, P. E. S., & McGuire, M. B. (1991). *Health, illness, and the social body*. Englewood Cliffs, NJ: Prentice Hall.
2. Ineichen, B. (1993). *Homes and health: How housing and health interact*. London: E & FN.
3. Ibid.
4. Duvall, D., & Booth, A. (1978). The housing environment and women's health. *Journal of Health & Social Behavior*, 19 (December), 410-417.
5. Ibid.
6. Ineichen, B. (1993).
7. Housing Preservation and Development. (1991). *Housing and vacancy report: New York City 1991*. (Source: U.S. Bureau of the Census Housing and Vacancy Report). New York: City of New York, p. 51.
8. Ibid, p. 56.
9. Ineichen, B. (1993).
10. Ibid, p. 54.
11. Stokols, D., & Shumaker, S. A. (1982). The psychological context of residential mobility and well-being. *Journal of Social Issues*, 38 (3), p. 151.
12. Ibid, p. 150.
13. Ibid, p. 154.
14. Wolfe, S., & Badgley, R. (1972). Patients and their families. *Milbank Memorial Fund Quarterly*, 50, Part II (2), 69-89.
15. Poland, B. D., Taylor, M. S., & Hayes, M. V. (1990). The ecology of health services utilization in Grenada, West Indies. *Social Science Medicine*, 30 (1), 13-24.
16. Fowler, M. G., Simpson, G. A., & Schoendorf, K. C. (1993). Families on the move and children's health care. *Pediatrics*, 91 (5), 934-940.
17. Weitzman, B. C., Knickman, J. R., & Shinn, M. (1990). Pathways to homelessness among New York City families. *Journal of Social Issues*, 46 (4), 125-140.
18. Ibid.
19. Ibid, p. 136.
20. Ibid, p. 133.

NOTES

CHAPTER 2

The Poverty Connection between Homelessness and Health

In the beginning of his first term, President Clinton declared the "end of welfare as we know it." Later in the term, Congress passed legislation establishing time limits and other restrictions on entitlements to public assistance. The Urban Institute has estimated that over one million more children will move into the ranks of poverty, as a result of the new policy. Advocates for the poor claim this legislation will lead to increased homelessness and more uninsured families.[1] Future research will determine their prescience. Even without radical changes to welfare, incremental changes over the years have made homelessness a more common consequence of poverty.

POVERTY AND HOMELESSNESS

In a nationwide telephone survey, Link, et al. found that 20 percent of people who were ever on welfare had been literally homeless—on the streets or in shelter—during their lifetime.[2] This was true for only 3 percent of those who had never received public assistance. Nationwide, families are the fastest growing group of the homeless population.[3] In New York City, the number of homeless families in shelter began climbing in the early 1980s, peaking at 5200 families in 1988.[4] After a decline for several years, the count peaked again at 5200 homeless families in 1992, with close to 1000 new families entering the city's shelter system each month. Today, 4500 families, including 7700 children, reside in city shelters on any given night.[5] This lower count may reflect a combination of an improved economy and the concerted efforts by the current city administration to divert families requesting shelter to alternative housing arrangements, through their existing social networks, when caseworkers can determine that such alternatives are available.[6]

POVERTY AND HEALTH

Poverty is perpetuated by the friction between the labor market and the family system: low wage jobs, lasting unemployment, homes without fathers, economic and educational discrimination and chronic impairments.[7] Family homelessness represents an extreme case of poverty, even if it is mostly a temporary situation.[8] Not surprisingly, researchers have found that homeless families face greater exposure to health risks and psycho-social problems, and more challenges in accessing health care compared to the general population.[9,10,11] Rafferty and Shinn suggest that exposure to poor nutrition, crowding, poor sanitation and high noise levels—all risks to well-being—may be more likely during an episode of homelessness.[12] Unfortunately, such risks are also common conditions of urban poverty.[13–16]

Compared to those of higher socioeconomic class, poor adults and children are more likely to experience malnutrition and obesity, live in crowded, unsanitary conditions and polluted environments, and engage in health-risky behaviors such as smoking and drinking.[17] When adjusted for health status, families living in poverty conditions have fewer physician visits, receive less preventive care, and are more likely to use hospital clinics and less likely to use private physicians' offices than more affluent families.[18–21] Poor families have greater health care needs compared to higher-income families; they also have more difficulty gaining appropriate access to health care services.[22–26]

HOMELESSNESS AND HEALTH

In contrast to health comparisons with the general population, homeless families look quite similar to poor families who are housed; both groups report a high degree of chronic health problems. In comparing poor, housed families on public assistance with welfare families entering shelter (many for their first shelter stay), Knickman, et al. found that chronic health problems such as asthma, bronchitis, high blood pressure and anemia were common among mothers of both groups.[27] The Stanford Center found no differences in health status between housed, poor children and homeless children living in shelter in the San Francisco area; ear problems, eye problems, asthma and musculo-skeletal disorders were common chronic health problems.[28] In Boston, 15 percent of mothers in shelter and 19 percent of poor, housed mothers reported that their children suffered from medical illnesses that required ongoing medical attention.[29] Homeless children sampled from a public hospital outpatient clinic in New York had similar rates of chronic illness as their domiciled counterparts.[30]

Most research on homeless children is based on a convenience sampling of children staying in emergency shelter.[31] Children living in public places may face greater health risks. The Stanford Center found that 14 percent of families who had lived in "inappropriate places, such as garages, outdoors, cars and empty public buildings," had a chronic illness, compared with 5 percent for other homeless children who had never lived in these settings.[32] Street-living is an extreme but atypical form of family homelessness in New York City. With regard to health and other conditions of well-being, street-homelessness may very well be distinguishable from living in shelter.

Nonetheless, there is little evidence to suggest that homeless families living in shelter suffer more from chronic health problems compared to other poor, domiciled families. Likewise, there is little evidence to suggest that health problems are a significant cause of family homelessness.[33] As with other conditions of poverty, chronic health problems among homeless families are likely to have predated their homelessness.

HIV/AIDS is a specific chronic condition for which the prevalence among low-income, minority women has been well-reported. Today, there are more than 22,000 women (13 years and older) in New York City living with AIDS.[34] Blacks make up more than half (53%) of all cases of women with AIDS in New York City. Hispanic women make up another 32 percent. Among both black and Hispanic women, intravenous drug-use is responsible for 54 percent of the transmissions. Among Hispanic women, another 35 percent of transmissions are related to heterosexual contact; the same is true for 27 percent of black women. Blacks make up over 75 percent of pediatric AIDS cases as well. [35]

However, very little data have been published regarding HIV infection among homeless mothers and families.[36] Findings of a link are mainly anecdotal.[37] In a study of minority women residing in homeless shelters and drug recovery programs, intravenous drug use, a high risk-factor for contracting HIV, was most prevalent among high-acculturated Latinas, whereas high-risk sexual activity was most prevalent among African-American women.[38]

Mothers who become homeless are clearly a subset of the population of poor, minority women who are at significant risk for HIV infection.[39] Whether homelessness further increases this risk is unknown, since there are no published studies comparing HIV infection rates of homeless mothers to that of poor, housed women. Nattell and Pulver found an 11 percent HIV prevalence rate among pregnant women living in shelters in New York City, but there was no comparison group.[40] Prevalence was highest for Latinas (15%) and women 35 years of age and older (21%).

PREVENTIVE CARE AND THE UTILIZATION GAP FOR HOMELESS FAMILIES

There is considerable evidence that compared to other poor families, homeless families, particularly children, under-utilize preventive care services, such as immunizations, and fare worse on outcomes which are related to a lack of prenatal and preventive care, such as infant mortality, low birth weight and lead poisoning.[41] Put another way, homeless families tend to look worse off than poor, housed families, based on quantitative measures of preventive care and related health outcomes made by medical providers.

In comparing medical records of homeless children seen at a New York City clinic, with those of housed, poor children also seen at the clinic, Alperstein, Rappaport and Flanigan found that 27 percent of homeless children and only 8 percent of housed children had delays in meeting immunization schedules.[42] Homeless children had elevated levels of lead in their system, higher hospital admission rates, and more reports of child abuse or neglect. With regard to child development, which is highly affected by diet and nutrition, they found no differences in rates of below normal height and weight. A more recent study, which evaluated children under five years of age at an inner city clinic, found that those who had been homeless in the previous year tended to be slightly shorter but did not weigh less.[43] Homeless children also were more likely to be hospitalized and saw health care providers more frequently.

In the Stanford Center studies, immunization rates among homeless and housed children under six years of age varied much less.[44] Eighteen percent of homeless children, 16 percent of "at-risk" children and 12 percent of formerly homeless children were behind in their immunization schedules. More troubling is that each of these groups of poor families had much higher non-compliance rates compared to the national average of only 3 percent.

In extreme contrast, however, Bassuk, Rubin and Lauriat reported in their study of 80 homeless families and 151 children in the Boston area that "only one child had not received his inoculations."[45] Parenthetically, many of the findings from the Bassuk group's sample of homeless families paint a very different picture from those found in other studies. Perhaps they reflect measurement differences or programs and policies unique to that area of study.

In an ethnographic study of 15 homeless mothers with children residing in the Detroit metropolitan area, "mothers acknowledged that keeping immunization shots current would have to be delayed until permanent housing was obtained."[46] Women's preoccupation with finding permanent housing left little time or energy for providing children with on going health care, according to researchers. None of the three pregnant women who were interviewed had yet obtained prenatal care. Women felt they could not get medical attention for themselves until they were permanently housed.

A New York City study of families in "welfare" hotels found that 40 percent of homeless women who gave birth received no prenatal care, compared with about 15 percent of a poor, housed comparison group. During the same study period, only nine percent of all women in New York City gave birth without prenatal care.[47] Rates of low-birth weight babies were higher for homeless mothers than housed mothers (16% v. 11%). More striking is the higher infant mortality rate of 25 deaths per 1000 live births for homeless women, compared to an infant mortality rate of 17 for poor housed women and a rate of 9 for all of New York City. These findings represent the most alarming health care outcomes for homeless families. They are all the more so because of the strong association found between family homelessness and pregnancy or having recently given birth.[48,49] Unclear is whether these differences are evident before mothers enter shelter and whether they persist after mothers leave shelter.

HOSPITALIZATION

The United Hospital Fund's study on children's hospitalization rates in New York City showed that children from the poorest neighborhoods had the highest levels of hospitalization for illnesses (otitis media, bronchitis and upper respiratory infections) that are usually treated or managed in an ambulatory setting.[50] Differences by income, in neighborhood hospitalization rates for conditions sensitive to ambulatory care intervention, have also been found for adults. We do not know to what extent homeless families accounted for these outcomes. However, Billings, et al. found that some of the city's "most notorious welfare hotels" (which house homeless families) were concentrated in two ZIP code areas with very high pediatric hospitalization rates.[51] In another New York City study, the overall hospitalization rate for children living in welfare hotels was 11.6 per 1000, compared to 7.5 per 1000 for a comparison group of children living in the same health district.[52]

Researchers of the United Hospital Fund studies concluded that a number of enabling factors contributed to differences in the hospitalization rates. A lack of primary care resources in poor neighborhoods; higher levels and severity of illness among low-income families because of conditions of poverty; and differences between physician practice patterns in hospital-based settings and private office or clinic settings were cited as the most plausible explanations for the gradient in hospitalization rates by neighborhood income levels.[53,54] Household income by geographical area explained more than 70 percent of the variation in rates.

EMERGENCY CARE

Emergency room use makes up a small portion of all health care visits in the general population, yet those *without* a regular source of care use emergency rooms at higher rates than those *with* a regular source of care.[55] Wood and Valdez reported that homeless families in Los Angeles were much less likely to report having a regular provider for sick care compared with poor housed families (72% v. 95%).[56] They also reported that families living in shelter were more likely than housed poor families to use emergency departments and clinics rather than private offices for both preventive care (35% v. 15%) and sick care (37% v. 26%).

Fine, et al. found that homeless children living in New York City's family shelters accounted for 9 percent of all children's emergency department visits over a one-year period.[57] It is unclear as to what portion of visits were made by all poor children. Homeless children were admitted from the emergency department at slightly higher rates than domiciled children (10% v. 8%, respectively). The finding suggests that homeless children may experience more acute problems than children in the general population, but not necessarily more than other *poor* children experience. In the Stanford Center study, homeless children did not have higher rates of acute illnesses compared to poor, housed children.[58]

THE ROLE OF MEDICAID

The "market" approach of Medicaid was intended to enable the poor to express their demand for health care services, which would then attract a supply of providers to meet this demand.[59] However, by some accounts, Medicaid, instead, had the unintended effect of shifting utilization from private physicians to publicly funded institutions.[60] The combination of a lack of health resources—in urban areas especially—and low Medicaid reimbursement to physicians, in general, have helped to keep many poor communities medically underserved. While insurance coverage significantly increases the likelihood of having a regular source of care at all,[61] these conditions also reinforced the structure of a dual medical care system: the privately insured using private sources and the publicly insured using public institutions.[62–64] The latter are considered to be less likely to provide preventive services and offer a continuity of care, which are important quality issues in the management of chronic illnesses. In one study, patients who used hospital outpatient departments as a regular source of care were found to see the same doctor on a repeated basis only half as often as patients who regularly obtained care at private offices.[65]

Nonetheless, Medicaid coverage has been widely shown to improve poor families' access to health care.[66–69] Newacheck and Halfron found that among children in fair or poor health, middle- and high-income children averaged 10 and 10.5 physician visits annually, while low-income children with Medicaid averaged 9.3 annual visits.[70] Low-income children in poor health and without Medicaid fared worst, averaging only 7.7 visits annually.

Despite almost thirty years of publicly sponsored health insurance for the poor, and along with it, overall improvements in access to a regular source of care, equity in the utilization of health services, based on need, is far from being achieved, much less equity in health status itself. Indeed, while the gap between utilization of physician services has declined over the last thirty years, the poor are still much more likely to have activity limitations due to health problems compared to the non-poor .[71]

Gaps in coverage and access among minority populations are well-documented.[72–76] Homeless families also tend to fall into a Medicaid coverage gap. For example, Miller and Lin found that for a sample of 158 homeless children in Kings County, Washington, only 40 percent were covered by Medicaid and 35 percent had no health insurance; 59 percent of the homeless children had no regular source of health care.[77] Bass, et al. found that 58 percent of the 78 children entering a family shelter located near Boston were "medically homeless" (had no regular source of care), even though the majority were eligible for Medicaid, and some even had private insurance.[78]

Wood, et al. found that 43 percent of homeless families had their welfare benefits discontinued during the last year, while only 23 percent of housed, poor families had ever seen their case closed.[79] In a nationwide study on homelessness, only 33 percent of women with children reported receiving public assistance income during the thirty days before their interview.[80] In a 16-city study of homelessness, Wright and Weber found that slightly more than half (55%) of homeless women were receiving any form of public assistance.[81] One-quarter of these women were estimated to have dependent children in their care. In great contrast to these findings, however, Bassuk, et al. reported that 91 percent of families were receiving public assistance at the time they were interviewed in emergency shelter.[82]

Findings from a growing body of literature suggest that public health insurance coverage is necessary but not sufficient to ensure appropriate utilization of health care services by poor families[83–87] and homeless adults.[88] These findings also suggest that Medicaid coverage appears to be an important factor to consider in examining the relationship between homelessness and health care utilization among poor families. However, the nature of this relationship may vary by geographical area because each state has flexibility in setting income thresholds for welfare eligibility and determining the scope of

Medicaid-covered health care services. Of significant concern is to what extent more stringent rules on entitlement to public assistance—through welfare reform—may lead more economically disadvantaged families into homelessness, and increase their risk of losing Medicaid coverage, which may then (further) hinder their access to health care.

LIMITATIONS OF CROSS-SECTIONAL STUDIES

Our understanding of the effects of homelessness on health care utilization has been limited, in part, because longitudinal data are needed to untangle the time-order of events and behavior. Only a few longitudinal studies have been conducted which included homeless families[89,90,91] or families who use public assistance.[92–94] To date, none has compared both groups over time, and none has specifically looked at health care utilization.

Most studies on family homelessness examine families at one point in time, typically during a current stay in shelter,[95–98] making it difficult to untangle whether the conditions or outcomes observed preceded or followed homelessness. Those who are homeless for longer periods of time stand a higher probability of being selected at random compared to those with shorter episodes of homelessness.[99] Thus, findings from cross-sectional studies are biased towards long-term shelter users, who may account for the bulk of shelter days, but may not represent the majority of homeless families. This limitation must be kept in mind, in reviewing findings from cross-sectional studies presented in the next chapter.

NOTES

1. Zedlewski, S., Clark, S., Meier, E., & Watson, K. (1996). *Potential effects of congressional welfare reform legislation on family incomes.* Washington, DC: The Urban Institute.

2. Link, B. G., Susser, E., Stueve, A., Phelan, J., Moore, R. E., & Struening, E. (1994). Lifetime and five-year prevalence of homelessness in the United States. *American Journal of Public Health*, 84 (12), 1907-1912.

3. Fantasia, R., & Isserman, M. (1994). *Homelessness: A sourcebook.* New York: Facts on File, Inc.

4. Homes for the Homeless. (1992). A generation of homeless families. *The New Poverty* (June), pp. 1-7.

5. Holloway, L. (1998, February 8). City asks an earlier verdict on shelter eviction rules. *The New York Times*, p. 37.

6. Department of Homeless Services. (1998). *Services at the department of homeless services*. New York: City of New York.

7. Muller, C. (1986). Review of twenty years of research on medical care utilization. *Health Services Research*, 21 (2), 129-144.

8. Shinn, M., & Weitzman, B. C. (1996). Homeless families are different. In J. Baumohl (Ed.), *Homelessness in America: A reference book* (pp. 109-122). New York: Oryx Press.

9. Brickner, P. W., Scharer-Keen L., Conanan, B., Elvy, A., & Savarese, M. (1985). *Health care of homeless people*. New York: Springer Publishing Company.

10. Institute of Medicine. (1988). *Homelessness, health and human needs*. Washington, DC: National Academy Press.

11. Molnar, J. M., Rath, W. R., & Klein. (1990). Constantly compromised: The impact of homelessness on children. *Journal of Social Issues*, 46 (4), 109-124.

12. Rafferty, Y., & Shinn, M. (1991). The Impact of homelessness on children. *American Psychologist*, 46 (11), 1170-1179.

13. Banta, H. D. (1990). What is health care? In A. R. Kovner (Ed.), *Health care delivery in the United States* (4th ed., pp. 8-30), New York: Springer Publishing Company.

14. Freund, P. E. S., & McGuire, M. B. (1991). *Health, illness, and the social body*. Englewood Cliffs, NJ: Prentice Hall.

15. Kleinman, J. C., Gold, M., & Makuc, D. (1981). Use of ambulatory medical care by the poor: Another look at equity. *Medical Care*, 19 (10), 1011-1029.

16. Wan, T. T. H., & Soifer, S. J. (1974). Determinants of physician utilization: A causal analysis. *Journal of Health & Social Behavior*, 15 (June), 100-107.

17. Freund, P. E. S., & McGuire, M. B. (1991).

18. Dutton, D. B. (1978). Explaining the low use of health services by the poor: Costs, attitudes, or delivery systems? *American Sociological Review*, 43 (6), 348-368.

19. McKinlay, J. B. (1975). The health-seeking behavior of the poor. In J. Kosa, & I. K. Zola (Eds.), *Poverty and health: A sociological analysis* (pp. 224-273). Cambridge, MA: Harvard University Press.

20. Muller, C. (1986). Review of twenty years of research on medical care utilization. *Health Services Research*, 21 (2), 129-144.

21. Newacheck, P. W., & Butler, L. H. (1983). Patterns of physician use among low-income, chronically ill persons. *Medical Care*, 21 (10), 981-989.

22. Freund, P. E. S., & McGuire, M. B. (1991).

23. Bazzoli, G. J. (1986). Health care for the indigent: Overview of critical issues. *Health Services Research*, 21(3), 353-402.

24. Kleinman, J. C., Gold, M., & Makuc, D. (1981). Use of ambulatory medical care by the poor: Another look at equity. *Medical Care*, 19 (10), 1011-1029.

25. Szapiro, N. (1988). Children, poverty, and hospital care in New York City. In M. I. Krasner (Ed.), *Poverty and health in New York City* (pp. 81-101). New York: United Hospital Fund.

26. Wolfe, B. L. (1980). Children's utilization of medical care. *Medical Care*, 18 (12), 1196-1207.

27. Knickman, J. R., Weitzman, B. C., Shinn M., & Marcus, E. H. (1989). *A study of homeless families in New York City: Characteristics and comparisons with other public assistance families* (Final Report: Volume 2). New York: New York University, Health Research Program.

28. The Stanford Center for the Study of Families, Children & Youth. (1991). *The nine studies of homeless families, children and youth.* Stanford, CA: Author.

29. Bassuk, E. L., & Rosenberg, L. (1990). Psychosocial characteristics of homeless children and children with homes. *Pediatrics*, 85 (3), 257-261.

30. Fierman, A. H., Dreyer, B. P., Quinn, L., Shulman, S., Courtlandt, C., & Guzzo, R. (1991). Growth delay in homeless children. *Pediatrics*, 88 (5), 918-925.

31. Rafferty, Y., & Shinn, M. (1991).

32. The Stanford Center for the Study of Families, Children & Youth. (1991).

33. Knickman, J. R., Weitzman, B. C., Shinn M., & Marcus, E. H. (1989).

34. New York State Department of Health. (1998, March). HIV/AIDS quarterly updates (Table 2 B). Albany, NY: Author.

35. Office of AIDS Surveillance. (1994). *AIDS surveillance update, 4th Quarter 1993.* New York: City of New York, Department of Health.

36. Fischer, P. J., & Breakey, W. R. (1991). The epidemiology of alcohol, drug, and mental disorders among homeless persons. *American Psychologist*, 46 (11), 1115-1128.

37. Singer, M. (1994). AIDS and the health crisis of the U.S. urban poor: The perspective of critical medical anthropology. *Social Science Medicine*, 39 (7), 931-947.

38. Nyamathi, A., Bennett, C., Leake, B., Lewis, C. & Flaskerud, J. (1993). AIDS-related knowledge, perceptions, and behaviors among impoverished minority women, *American Journal of Public Health*, 83 (1), 65-71.

39. Weeks, M. R., Schensul, J. J., Williams, S. S., Singer M., & Grier, M. (1995). AIDS prevention for African-American and Latina women: Building culturally and gender-appropriate intervention. *AIDS Education & Prevention*, 7 (3), 251-264.

40. Nattell, T., Pulver, W. (1996, October). *HIV prevalence among pregnant homeless women served by a mobile prenatal care clinic in New York City*. Paper presented at the meeting of the American Public Health Association, New York, NY.

41. Burg, M. A. (1994). Health problems of sheltered homeless women and their dependent children. *Health & Social Work*, 19 (2), 125-131.

42. Alperstein, G., Rappaport, C., & Flanigan, J. M. (1988). Health problems of homeless children in New York City. *American Journal of Public Health*, 78 (9), 1232-1233.

43. Cutts, D.B., Pheley, A.M., & Geppert, J.S. (1996, October). *Profile of young children with a history of homelessness receiving care at an inner-city hospital clinic*. Paper presented at the meeting of the American Public Health Association, New York, NY.

44. The Stanford Center for the Study of Families, Children & Youth. (1991).

45. Bassuk, E. L., Rubin, L., & Lauriat, A. S. (1986). Characteristics of sheltered homeless families. *American Journal of Public Health*, 76 (9), p. 1100.

46. Thrasher, S. P., & Mowbray, C. T. (1995). A strengths perspective: An ethnographic study of homeless women with children. *Health & Social Work*, 20 (5), p. 98.

47. Chavkin, W., Kristal, A., Seabron, C., & Guigli, P. E. (1987). Reproductive experiences of women living in hotels for the homeless in New York City. *New York State Journal of Medicine*, 87, 10-13.

48. Weitzman, B. C. (1989). Pregnancy and childbirth: Risk factors for homelessness? *Family Planning Perspectives*, 21 (4), 175-178.

49. Wiecha, J. L., Dwyer, J. T., & Dunn-Strohecker, M. (1991). Nutrition and health services needs among the homeless. *Public Health Reports*, 106 (4), 364-373.

50. Szapiro, N. (1988).

51. Billings, J., Zeitel, L., Lukomnik, J., Carey, T. S., Blank, A. E., & Newman, L. (1993). Impact of socioeconomic status on hospital use in New York City. *Health Affairs*, 12, p. 170.

52. Alperstein, G., Rappaport, C., & Flanigan, J. M. (1988).

53. Billings, et al. (1993).

54. Szapiro, N. (1988).

55. Orr, S. T., Charney, E., Straus, J., & Bloom, B. (1991). Emergency room use by low income children with a regular source of health care. *Medical Care*, 29 (3), 283-286.

56. Wood, D., & Valdez, R. B. (1991). Barriers to medical care for homeless families compared with housed poor families. *American Journal of Diseases of Children*, 145 (10), 1109-1115.

57. Fine, J., Foltin, G., Tunik, M., Fierman, A., & Dreyer, B. (1990). Ambulance utilization by homeless children. *American Journal of Childhood Diseases*, 144 (April), 433.

58. The Stanford Center for the Study of Families, Children & Youth. (1991).

59. Dutton, D. B. (1978). Explaining the low use of health services by the poor: Costs, attitudes, or delivery systems? *American Sociological Review*, 43 (6), 348-368.

60. Orr, S. T., Charney, E., Straus, J., & Bloom, B. (1991).

61. Lewin-Epstein, N. (1991). Determinants of regular source of health care in Black, Mexican, Puerto Rican, and Non-Hispanic white populations. *Medical Care*, 29 (6), 543-557.

62. Braveman, P., Bennett, T., Lewis, C., Egerter, S., & Showstack, J. (1993). Access to prenatal care following major Medicaid eligibility expansions. *JAMA*, 269 (March 10), 1285-1289.

63. Dutton, D.B. (1978).

64. Rowland, D., & Salganicoff, A. (1994). Commentary: Lessons from Medicaid: Improving access to office-based physicians care for the low-income population. *American Journal of Public Health*, 84 (4), 550-552.

65. Newacheck, P. W., & Butler, L. H. (1983). Patterns of physician use among low-income, chronically ill persons. *Medical Care*, 21 (10), 981-989.

66. Ibid.

67. Guendelman, S., & Schwalbe, J. (1986). Medical care utilization by Hispanic children. *Medical Care*, 24 (10), 925-940.

68. Saver, B. G., & Peterfreund, N. (1993). Insurance, income, and access to ambulatory care in King County, Washington. *American Journal of Public Health*, 83 (11), 1583-1588.

69. Wells, K. B., Golding, J. M., Hough, R. L., Burnam, A., & Karno, M. (1988). Factors affecting the probability of use of general and medical health and social/community services for Mexican Americans and non-Hispanic whites. *Medical Care*, 26 (5), 441-452.

70. Newacheck, P.W., & Halfron, N. H. (1986). Access to Ambulatory Care Services for Economically Disadvantaged Children. *Pediatrics*, 87 (5), 813-818.

71. National Center for Health Statistics. (1992). *National Ambulatory Medical Care Survey 1989*, (series 13, No. 110) Washington, DC: U.S. Government Printing Office.

72. Cunningham, P. J., & Cornelius, L. J. (1995). Access to ambulatory care for American Indians and Alaska natives: The relative importance of personal and community resources. *Social Science Medicine*, 40 (3), 393-407.

73. Davis, K., & Rowland, D. (1991). Financing health care for the poor. In E. Ginzberg (Ed.), *Health Services Research* (pp. 93-125). Cambridge, MA: Harvard University Press.

74. General Accounting Office [GAO]. (1995). Uninsured and children on Medicaid (from Report No. GAO/HEHS-95-83R). *Medical Benefits*, 12 (8), 4.

75. Moore, P., & Hepworth, J. T. (1994). Use of perinatal and infant health services by Mexican-American Medicaid enrollees. *JAMA*, 272 (July 27), 297-404.

76. Rosenbaum, S., Hughes, D. C., & Johnson, K. (1988). Maternal and child health services for medically indigent children and pregnant women. *Medical Care*, 26 (4), 315-331.

77. Miller, D. S., & Lin, E. H. B. (1988). Children in sheltered homeless families: Reported health status and use of health services. *Pediatrics*, 81(5), 668-673.

78. Bass, J. L., Brennan, P., Mehta, K., & Kodzis, S. (1990). Pediatric problems in a suburban shelter for homeless families. *Pediatrics*, 85 (1), p. 37.

79. Wood, D., Valdez, R. B., Hayashi, T., & Shen, A. (1990). Homeless and housed families in Los Angeles: A study comparing demographic, economic, and family function characteristics. *American Journal of Public Health*, 80, 1049-1052.

80. Burt, M. R. (1992). *Over the edge: The growth of homelessness in the 1980s*. New York: Russell Sage Foundation.

81. Wright, J. D., & Weber, E. (1988). Determinants of benefit-program participation among the urban homeless. *Evaluation Review*, 12 (4), 376-395.

82. Bassuk, E. L., Rubin, L., & Lauriat, A. S. (1986).

83. Bashshur, R. L., Homan, R. K., & Smith, D. G. (1994). Beyond the uninsured: Problems in access to care. *Medical Care*, 32 (5), 409-419.

84. Carr, W., Cohen, S., Schop, J. A., & Rink, R. (1988). An unfinished agenda: Reducing the health deficit. In M. I. Krasner (Ed.), *Poverty and health in New York City* (pp. 21-47). New York: United Hospital Fund.

85. Institute of Medicine. (1988).

86. Newacheck, P.W., & Halfron, N. H. (1986).

87. Wolfe, B. L. (1980).

88. Padgett, D., Struening, E., & Andrews, H. (1990). Factors affecting the use of medical, mental health, alcohol, and drug treatment services by homeless adults. *Medical Care*, 28 (9), 805-821.

89. Culhane, D. P., Dejowski, E. F., Ibanez, J., Needham, E., & Macchia, I. (1993). *Public Shelter Admission Rates in Philadelphia and New York City.* Washington, DC: Office of Housing Research, Fannie Mae.

90. Sosin, M., Piliavin, I., & Westerfelt, H. (1990). Toward a longitudinal analysis of homelessness. *Journal of Social Issues*, 46 (4), 157-174.

91. Weitzman, B. C., Knickman, J. R., & Shinn, M. (1990). Pathways to homelessness among New York City families. *Journal of Social Issues*, 46 (4), 125-140.

92. Bane, M. J., & Ellwood, D. T. (1986). Slipping into and out of poverty: The dynamics of spells. *Inquiry*, 21 (Winter), 1-23.

93. Ashworth, K., Hill, M., & Walker, R. (1994). Patterns of childhood poverty: New challenges for policy. *Journal of Policy Analysis and Management*, 13 (4), 658-680.

94. Short, P. F., Cantor, J. C., & Monheit, A. C. (1988). The dynamics of Medicaid enrollment. *Inquiry*, 25 (Winter), 504-516.

95. Bassuk, E. L. (1991). Homeless families. *Scientific American*, 265 (December), 66-74.

96. Goodman, L. A. (1991). The relationship between social support and family homelessness: A comparison study of homeless and housed mothers. *Journal of Community Psychology*, 19 (October), 321-332.

97. Winkleby, M. A., & Boyce, W. T. (1994). Health-related risk factors of homeless families and single adults. *Journal of Community Health*, 19 (February), 7–23.

98. Wood, D. & Valdez, R. B. (1991).

99. Shinn, M. & Weitzman, B. C. (1996).

CHAPTER 3

A Profile of Homeless Families in Urban America

Growing interest in families as a specialization of research on homelessness has produced a number of studies from around the country that describe the characteristics of homeless families[1–5] and the structural and individual determinants of family homelessness.[6–10] Below, the characteristics of urban homeless families are described and compared to other populations. Comparisons are made in the context of demographic and socio-economic factors that are believed to be associated with health care use or health status, based on an extensive medical sociology literature over the last several decades.[11–16]

AGE

Homeless families are typically younger, on average, than their housed counterparts.[17,18] In the Knickman, et al. study of public assistance families requesting shelter in New York City, 44 percent of mothers were under age 25, compared to only 18 percent of housed families on public assistance.[19] The average age for mothers on public assistance in Goodman's study of 100 families in the Boston area was 26.8 for homeless mothers, compared to 29.7 for housed mothers.[20] Mothers of families who become homeless tend to be in an earlier stage of their reproductive years compared to the overall population of mothers receiving public assistance.

GENDER AND ETHNICITY

The rise in homeless families has occurred amidst a steady rise in single-parent families since the early 1970s.[21] Both groups are over-represented by minorities, relative to their share of the population. Female headed households account for approximately 40 percent of the total population officially designated as poor. Almost half of all African-American and more than 40 percent of Hispanic children live in such households. According to the 1990 U.S. Census, black households make up about 27 percent of households receiving public assistance in New York City, but make up less than 16 percent of all New York City households.

The vast majority of homeless families are headed by single women; 80 percent are non-white.[22] In New York City, blacks are disproportionately represented among homeless families. In the Knickman, et al. study, 54 percent of randomly selected families requesting shelter were black, while only 32 percent of a random sample of housed families on public-assistance were black. Puerto Ricans made up 33 percent of shelter requesters and 41 percent of housed families on public assistance.[23] New York City, as a whole, is 24 percent Hispanic.[24] African-American and Hispanic families also make up the largest ethnic groups of homeless families in the San Francisco Bay area[25] and in other urban areas.[26]

MARRIAGE

Mixed findings have been reported on marital status, which may be related, in part, to policies that exclude men from shelter or from shelter counts.[27] Most studies have found that a low percentage of homeless mothers are married: 8 percent;[28] 10 percent;[29] 18 percent;[30] 30 percent.[31] Knickman, et al. found that New York City's homeless mothers were more likely to report being married (or living with someone) than poor, housed mothers (23% v. 9%).[32] Shinn and Weitzman hypothesized that this finding may reflect welfare policies that create disincentives for housed mothers to report being married.[33] At the same time, some shelters may exclude men or require them to give evidence of marriage or paternity before being admitted as a family. Thus, such policies may give homeless families an incentive to report being married or living with someone.

FAMILY SIZE AND COMPOSITION

Differences in the number of children a mother has ever had vary little between homeless and housed poor families.[34–36] On the other hand, homeless families tend to have fewer children with them. Knickman, et al. found that among those ages 26 through 30, both shelter-requesting and housed mothers, on average, had had about two children in their lifetime. At the time of being interviewed, the average number of children under 18 who were in their mother's custody was 1.6 for shelter requesters and 2.2 for housed mothers.[37]

Homelessness itself may be related to family separation. In some cases, shelters exclude men or adolescent boys, as mentioned earlier.[38] A mother may also voluntarily choose to leave children with other relatives or friends before entering shelter, or a social services agency may remove children from a family some time during the course of homelessness. In a study from the same sample analyzed for the research in this book, children from homeless families made up 85 percent of all children absent from their family at the time of the mother's follow up interview.[39] In addition, homeless children may be at greater risk for foster care placement. More than one-third of a random sample of foster care children, ages birth to three, had a biological parent who had been homeless.[40]

Family size, however, may also be related to the duration of homelessness. Knickman, et al. reported that large families experienced longer stays of homelessness once they entered shelter.[41] Affordable housing was harder to come by for larger families. However, family size did not increase the risk of becoming homeless.

A mother's child-custody status is highly associated with her profile as a homeless woman. Johnson and Krueger subdivided their sample of homeless mothers into those with their children and those without their children.[42] Mothers without their children were older, homeless longer, and were more likely to have a history of alcohol problems and treatment for mental illness. In a survey of women residing in New York City adult shelters, 75 percent were found to be mothers.[43] Forty percent were separated from dependent children under the age of 16.

EDUCATION AND EMPLOYMENT

Findings on levels of education achievement and work experience among homeless families are mixed. In general, mothers of homeless and housed poor families both have low educational attainment and weak employment histories.[44,45] For female heads of households on public assistance, neither a high school diploma, or equivalent, nor job experience protected poor families against homelessness.[46] Bassuk and Rosenberg[47] found that homeless families in the Boston area had higher levels of education than a housed comparison group, while the opposite was true in the Wood, et al.[48] study of homeless families in Los Angeles.

MENTAL ILLNESS

The homeless studies by Burt and Cohen concluded that homeless women with children have fewer mental health problems than homeless single women or single men.[49] In New York City, only 4 percent of homeless mothers requesting shelter reported ever having been hospitalized for mental illness, compared to only 1 percent for a comparison group of housed mothers on public assistance.[50] Studies of homeless female heads of households have found self-reported mental hospitalization rates ranging from 6 to 14 percent.[51] The low prevalence of severe mental illness (as measured by overnight stays in a mental hospital), among both the domiciled and recently homeless public assistance population, suggests that mental illness is not a significant cause of homelessness among families. However, for the very small number who reported it, mental hospitalization was a risk factor for becoming homeless.

Mental hospitalization tends to represent treatment for extreme psychiatric disorders. Low hospitalization rates do not reflect the prevalence of milder psychiatric disorders, which tend to be treated on an outpatient basis.[52] Weitzman, Knickman and Shinn found that about the same percentage (7%) of shelter requesters and their housed counterparts reported using a counselor/therapist or mental health clinic within the last year.[53] Their findings showed that neither the use of outpatient mental health services nor the use of prescription drugs for "nervous" problems was a significant risk factor for homelessness.

A study examining the influence of maternal psychosocial factors on pediatric service use found no evidence that maternal substance abuse, depression or low social support influenced the volume of physician visits for poor, urban children under five years of age.[54] These findings contrasted with those from other studies based on socio-economically representative samples of mothers. The researchers concluded that for women living in poverty, other factors, including single parent status, frequent moves and homelessness, may have a more direct effect on their children's utilization of pediatric services.

SUBSTANCE USE AND ABUSE

The Interagency Council on Homelessness claims that "substance abuse is an important factor in the 'selection' of homeless people from among others who are also poor."[55] Among homeless women with children, however, estimated rates of substance abuse (including alcohol and various types of illicit drugs), as with mental illness, are consistently less than rates for homeless single women or men.[56,57,58] Nonetheless, studies of mothers already in shelter find higher rates of substance use. Fierman, et al. found that of mothers presenting children for health care at a hospital clinic, 29 percent of homeless mothers and 7 percent of domiciled mothers reported past or present use of cocaine or heroin.[59] Bassuk and Rosenberg reported that 10 percent of female heads of homeless families in Boston were diagnosed as a substance abuser compared to less than 3 percent of a housed comparison group.[60]

Knickman, et al. found that mothers with a substance abuse problem were at greater risk for becoming homeless.[61] However, the proportion of mothers entering shelter who indicated a substance abuse problem was very small, which led researchers to conclude that substance abuse does not appear to be a major cause of homelessness among poor families.[62]

On a related note, the main reason that poor women are incarcerated is for drug-related charges.[63] Incarceration, itself, may lead women to lose contact with or custody of their children, while putting women at risk of becoming homeless, upon being released back into the community.

PSYCHO-SOCIAL FACTORS AND THEIR RELATIONSHIP TO HOMELESSNESS AND HEALTH CARE USE

In summary, the literature suggests that homeless mothers who have custody of their children are significantly better adjusted psycho-socially than single homeless women, and have rates of mental illness similar to those for poor housed mothers. There is evidence, however, that homeless mothers are more likely to have or have had a substance abuse problem. The research findings suggest that neither mental illness nor substance abuse is a major factor in the cause of *family* homelessness.

Mental illness and substance abuse are, however, conditions that may interfere with a mother's health care decision-making for herself or her children, or affect the need for health care among family members. An extensive literature on family systems theory, which has evolved from research in the fields of social work, family medicine and sociology, describes and explains the importance of family roles, functions, and structures on health status, and health care decision-making by and for family members.[64–71]

The studies, however, have focused mostly on middle class families, for which comparisons to low-income or poorly educated families may not apply. For example, a number of general population studies have found an indirect relationship between maternal depression and child health care use.[72] Yet, in a study of inner-city poor families with pre-school age children, neither maternal depression nor other psycho-social factors, including substance abuse, predicted emergency room visits, injury visits or delays in immunizations.[73] They suggested that psycho-social factors such as maternal depression and substance abuse may have more influence on making any contact with the health care system than on the total amount of utilization, once making initial contact with the system. Even among homeless adults, the relationship between mental health and health care utilization is weak. Padgett, Struening and Andrews found that mental health status was unrelated to the use of medical services among homeless adults.[74] Among poor families, other conditions of poverty—such as homelessness—may play a more important role in health care use than mental health and substance abuse. Thus, while psycho-social factors may put a small segment of families at risk of homelessness, they do not necessarily play a significant role in families' health care seeking behavior.

NOTES

1. Bassuk, E. L., Weinreb, L. F., Buckner, J. C., Browne, A., Salomon, A., & Bassuk, S. S. (1996). The characteristics and needs of sheltered homeless and low-income housed mothers. *JAMA*, 276 (August 28), 640-646.

2. Knickman, J. R., Weitzman, B. C., Shinn M., & Marcus, E. H. (1989). *A study of homeless families in New York City: Characteristics and comparisons with other public assistance families* (Final Report: Volume 2). New York: New York University, Robert F. Wagner Graduate School of Public Service, Health Research Program.

3. Wood, D., Valdez, R. B., Hayashi, T., & Shen, A. (1990). Homeless and housed families in Los Angeles: A study comparing demographic, economic, and family function characteristics. *American Journal of Public Health*, 80, 1049-1052.

4. Smith, E. M., & North, C. S. (1994). Not all homeless women are alike: Effects of motherhood and the presence of children. *Community Mental Health Journal*, 30 (6), 601-610.

5. Winkleby, M. A., & Boyce, W. T. (1994). Health-related risk factors of homeless families and single adults. *Journal of Community Health*, 19 (February), 7-23.

6. Dornbusch, S. M. (1994). Additional perspectives on homeless families. *American Behavioral Scientist*, 37 (3), 404-411.

7. Jacobs, F. H. (1994). Defining a social problem: the case of family homelessness. *American Behavioral Scientist*, 37 (3), 396-403.

8. Milburn, N., & D'Ercole, A. (1991). Homeless women: Moving toward a comprehensive model. *American Psychologist*, 46 (11), 1161-1169.

9. Molnar, J. M., Rath, W. R., & Klein. (1990). Constantly compromised: The impact of homelessness on children. *Journal of Social Issues*, 46 (4), 109-124.

10. Toro, P. A., Trickett, E. J., Wall, D. D., & Salem, D. A. (1991). Homelessness in the United States: An ecological perspective. *American Psychologist*, 46 (11), 1208-1218.

11. Aday, L. A. (1993). Indicators and predictors of health services utilization. In S. J. Williams, & P. R. Torrens (Eds.), *Introduction to Health Services* (4th ed., pp. 46-70). Albany, NY: Delmar Publishing, Inc.

12. McKinlay, J. B. (1975). The health-seeking behavior of the poor. In J. Kosa, & I. K. Zola (Eds.), *Poverty and health: A sociological analysis* (pp. 224-273). Cambridge, MA: Harvard University Press.

13. Markides, K. S., Levin, J. S., & Ray, L. A. (1985). Determinants of physician utilization among Mexican-Americans. *Medical Care*, 23 (3), 236-246.

14. Tanner, J. L., Cocherham, W. C., & Spaeth, J. L. (1983). Predicting physician utilization. *Medical Care*, 21 (3), 360-369.

15. Wan, T. T. H., & Soifer, S. J. (1974). Determinants of physician utilization: A causal analysis. *Journal of Health & Social Behavior*, 15 (June), 100-107.

16. Wells, K. B., Golding, J. M., Hough, R. L., Burnam, A., & Karno, M. (1988). Factors affecting the probability of use of general and medical health and social/community services for Mexican Americans and non-Hispanic whites. *Medical Care*, 26 (5), 441-452.

17. Rossi, P. H. (1994). Troubling Families: Family homelessness in America. *American Behavioral Scientist*, 37, 342-395.

18. Knickman, J.R., et al. (1989).

19. Ibid.

20. Goodman, L. A. (1991). The relationship between social support and family homelessness: A comparison study of homeless and housed mothers. *Journal of Community Psychology*, 19 (October), 321-332.

21. Interagency Council on the Homeless (1994). *Priority: Home!* Washington, DC: Author.

22. Interagency Council on the Homeless. (1991). *The 1990 annual report*. Washington, DC: Author.

23. Knickman, J. R., et al. (1989).

24. U.S. Census public use microdata files for New York City borough totals, 1990, as cited in Moss, M., Townsend A., Tobier, E. (1997, December). *Immigration is transforming New York City*. New York: New York University, Robert F. Wagner Graduate School of Public Service, Taub Urban Research Center.

25. The Stanford Center for the Study of Families, Children & Youth. (1991).

26. Fantasia, R., & Isserman, M. (1994). *Homelessness: A sourcebook*. New York: Facts on File, Inc.

27. Shinn, M., & Weitzman, B. C. (1996). Homeless families are different. In J. Baumohl (Ed.), *Homelessness in America: A reference book* (pp. 109-122). New York: Oryx Press.

28. Goodman, L. A. (1991).

29. Bassuk, E. L., Rubin, L., & Lauriat, A. S. (1986). Characteristics of sheltered homeless families. *American Journal of Public Health*, 76 (9), 1097-1101.

30. Burt, M. R. (1992). *Over the edge: The growth of homelessness in the 1980s*. New York: Russell Sage Foundation.

31. The Stanford Center. (1991).

32. Knickman, J.R., et al. (1989).

33. Shinn, M., & Weitzman, B. C. (1996).

34. Knickman, J. R., et al. (1989).

35. Goodman, L. A. (1991).

36. The Stanford Center. (1991).

37. Knickman, J. R., et al. (1989).

38. Shinn, M., & Weitzman, B. C. (1996).

39. Cowal, K., Shinn, M., & Stojanovic, D. (1996, October). *Parent-child separations among homeless and poor housed families in New York City*. Paper presented at the meeting of the American Public Health Association, New York, NY.

40. Zlotnick, C., Kronstadt, D., & Klee, L. (1996, October). *Foster care children, their parents and the cycle of homelessness*. Paper presented at the meeting of the American Public Health Association, New York, NY.

41. Knickman, J. R., et al. (1989).

42. Johnson, A. K., & Kreuger, L.W. (1989). Toward a better understanding of homeless women. *Social Work*, 34, 537-540.

43. Women's City Club of New York. (1992). *Beyond Facilities and Good Intentions*, New York: The Coalition for the Homeless.

44. Goodman, L. A. (1991).

45. Knickman, J. R., et al. (1989).

46. Ibid.

47. Bassuk, E. L., & Rosenberg, L. (1990). Psychosocial characteristics of homeless children and children with homes. *Pediatrics*, 85 (3), 257-261.

48. Wood, D., Valdez, R. B., Hayashi, T., & Shen, A. (1990).

49. Burt, M., & Cohen, B. (1989). Differences among homeless single women, women with children and single men. *Social Problems*, 35 (5), 508-524.

50. Knickman, J. R., et al. (1989).

51. Shinn, M., & Weitzman, B. C. (1996).

52. Fischer, P. J., & Breakey, W. R. (1991). The epidemiology of alcohol, drug, and mental disorders among homelessness persons. *American Psychologist*, 46 (11), 1115-1128.

53. Weitzman, B. C., Knickman, J. R., & Shinn, M. (1992). Predictors of shelter use among low-income families: Psychiatric history, substance abuse, and victimization. *American Journal of Public Health*, 82 (11), 1547-1550.

54. Watson, J. M., & Kemper, K. J. (1995). Maternal factors and children's health care use. *Social Science Medicine*, 40 (5), 623-628.

55. Interagency Council on the Homeless. (1994), p. 33.

56. Burt, M. R. (1992). *Over the edge: The growth of homelessness in the 1980s*. New York: Russell Sage Foundation.

57. Fischer, P. J., & Breakey, W. R. (1991).

58. Robertson, M. J. (1991). Homeless women with children: The role of alcohol and other drug abuse. *American Psychologist*, 46 (11), 1198-1204.

59. Fierman, A. H., Dreyer, B. P., Quinn, L., Shulman, S., Courtlandt, C., & Guzzo, R. (1991). Growth delay in homeless children. *Pediatrics*, 88 (5), 918-925.

60. Bassuk, E. L., & Rosenberg, L. (1990).

61. Knickman, J. R., et al. (1989).

62. Weitzman, B. C., Knickman, J. R., & Shinn, M. (1992).

63. J. Binney, Office of Correctional Health Services for the New York City Health and Hospitals Corporation, personal communication, November 18, 1996.

64. Counte, M. A., & Christman, L. P. (1981). *Interpersonal behavior and health care*. Boulder, CO: Westview Press.

65. Litman, T. J. (1974). The family as a basic unit in health and medical care: A social behavioral overview. *Social Science Medicine*, 8, 495-519.

66. Heller, P. L., Chalfant, H. P., Quesada, G. M., & Rivera-Worley, M. D. C. (1981). Class, familism and utilization of health services in Durango, Mexico: A replication. *Social Science Medicine*, 15A, 539-541.

67. Ell, K., & Northern, H. (1990). *Families and health care*. New York: Aldine de Gruyter.

68. Pratt, L. (1976). *Family structure and effective health behavior: The energized family*. Boston: Houghton Mifflin Co.

69. Litman, T. J., & Venters, M. (1979). Research on health care and the family: A methodological overview. *Social Science Medicine*, 13a, 379-385.

70. Montgomery, J., & Fewer, W. (1988). *Family systems and beyond*. New York: Human Sciences Press, Inc.

71. Eckert, J. K., & Goldstein, M. C. (1983). An anthropological approach to the study of illness behavior in an urban community. *Urban Anthropology*, 12 (2), 125-137.

72. Zuckerman, B. & Beardslee, W. R. (1987). Maternal depression: A concern for pediatricians. *Pediatrics*, 79, 110.

73. Watson, J. M., & Kemper, K. J. (1995).

74. Padgett, D., Struening, E., & Andrews, H. (1990). Factors affecting the use of medical, mental health, alcohol, and drug treatment services by homeless adults. *Medical Care*, 28 (9), 805-821.

CHAPTER 4

Design of the Study on Homeless and Housed Poor Families

RESEARCH QUESTIONS AND HYPOTHESES

Based on the findings reviewed in the literature, I developed three research questions regarding the relationship between residential instability and current patterns of health care use among poor, urban families:

I *Is residential mobility (independent of shelter use) associated with current patterns of health care use among poor families?*

A high degree of residential mobility often precedes entry into emergency shelter and may continue for the early years following it, making mobility an important aspect of residential instability. Whether recent episodes of residential mobility, or pre-shelter mobility are associated with homeless families' health care use has not been studied. Findings from studies on middle class individuals suggest that residential mobility is linked mainly with not having a regular source of care. Not having established a regular source of care is also associated with making no recent contact with the health care system. Because mobility has been so strongly linked with shelter use, and based on the findings of families living in shelter, I hypothesized that as the degree of mobility—either pre-shelter or post-shelter—increases, so does the likelihood of going without care. I hypothesized that the relative risk of using hospital and community clinic-based sources of care over private, office-based physicians increases as well. Because mobility's association with health status—a strong predictor of total health care use—is quite weak, I predicted that mobility would not be associated with the total volume of visits.

II *Is shelter use related to current patterns of health care use among poor families?*

As described in Chapter 2, studies have found that compared to poor, housed families, those living in shelter are more likely to use emergency departments and less likely to use private physicians. I hypothesized that having ever used shelter is related to poor families' current source of health care, controlling for their current housing situation and how long they lived in emergency housing. Based on what we know about the pathways to homelessness and family systems theory, it seems reasonable to expect that many homeless families, particularly those from multi-generational welfare families, and those who had never achieved their own household independence, may never have been well-integrated into the mainstream health care system.

The literature on homeless families has not reported on differences between homeless and housed families regarding the amount of medical care used. However, family homelessness is associated with an increased risk of losing public assistance. A lack of Medicaid coverage is associated with a greater likelihood of making no outpatient visits and with making fewer visits, on average. Therefore, I expected that shelter use would be associated with an increased likelihood of making no visits in the last year, and have a negative association with the total volume of annual medical visits.

III *Is the amount of time families spent in shelter associated with current patterns of health care use, among those who spent any time in shelter?*

The second set of hypotheses tacitly assumes that conditions related to becoming homeless, including factors of residential instability, may have shaped families' utilization of health care services, such that those patterns extend after shelter use. While not contradictory to the second set, the third set of hypotheses assumes that the experience of shelter use influences later health care use. The third research question addresses the long-term consequences of shelter use on health care utilization, based on the duration of homelessness. I predicted that "longer" shelter stays would have a greater association with utilization outcomes than "shorter" shelter stays. I expected that families who had longer stays in shelter were less likely to be currently using private sources of health care. Likewise, I hypothesized that a long shelter stay would be associated with a greater likelihood of making no visits in the last year, and would be associated with a decrease in the total number of annual medical visits.

A CONCEPTUAL MODEL FOR HEALTH CARE UTILIZATION

A large part of health services research is dedicated to examining how equitable a particular health care system is in providing access to care among various populations, as they differ by health status, income, race, and any number of other factors.[1] The Behavioral Model of Health Services Use,[2,3] first developed in the 1960s, is used in this research to examine health care use among poor families, as differentiated by their experiences with residential instability. Unfortunately, conceptual models of health care utilization have largely ignored residential instability as a factor in health care utilization. Ironically, Andersen and Newman included "residential mobility" as a predisposing factor of health care use in a graphical illustration of the Behavioral model, but they did not discuss how or why it might be related to utilization.[4] In fact, they never discussed it at all. Nonetheless, the model is arguably the most widely used conceptual framework for conducting health care utilization research, and is particularly noted for its application in studying health care use among families.[5]

Part of the popularity of the Behavioral model is that it is relatively simple to operationalize. It posits three sets of independent variables: predisposing, enabling and illness (or need), which influence different outcomes or patterns of health care use. These typically may include making any contact with the health care system over a given time period; the volume of outpatient visits and/or hospitalizations; having a regular source of care; and the type of care used on a regular basis.[6,7]

The model distinguishes individual factors, which are believed to have more to do with the likelihood of any use, from aspects of the health care system itself, which are considered more influential regarding where and how often a person seeks care.[8,9] Predisposing variables are individual characteristics which exist prior to specific episodes of illness occurring. They are empirically associated with various aspects of health and illness, and thus can influence use, but are not reasons for using health care per se. Predisposing variables are further delineated into demographic, social structural and health beliefs. Demographic characteristics include age, gender, marital status, and past illness. They represent proxy measures of different physiological and life-cycle states. Social structure factors are used as proxy measures of social position in society. These include ethnicity, education, occupation, family size, religion and residential mobility. There is general recognition that people with similar social backgrounds tend to emulate similar lifestyles that are reflected in health care utilization behavior; much less is known about *why* these variables matter.[10]

The model posits that enabling family and community factors enhance access to and use of health services. Family enabling factors typically include income, health insurance, and family size. In studies of vulnerable populations, welfare status, substance abuse, mental illness or other psycho-social factors may be included as enabling factors. In recent work on homeless single adults, the model was expanded to include subsistence needs, including housing.[11] Community enabling factors refer to levels of health care resources, such as physician-to-population ratios for a given geographical area. Hospital resources may be measured by the number of beds, or the proximity or presence within a geographical unit.

The need for health care services, whether perceived by an individual or evaluated by a clinician, is considered the most immediate reason for a person to seek health care. Self-reported health status, which is highly correlated with utilization, is a common measure of perceived need. Health utilization studies have consistently demonstrated that medical need, or illness level, is the strongest predictor of the volume of health care use.[12–14] While large surveys of national, representative samples, conducted by Andersen and colleagues in the 1970s explained only 16 to 25 percent of the variance in making contact with a physician and the volume of physician visits, from that yield, 85 percent of the variance was explained by perceived or evaluated health need variables.[15]

Such findings have led to criticism over the efficacy of the model in health care utilization studies.[16–19] The results suggest that our health care system is equitable if medical need and not enabling or predisposing variables are the main determinants of use. Yet, there is a wealth of evidence to show that access to health care is far from equitable for the many individuals who are disenfranchised from the health care system because of their skin color, lack of income or health insurance, or live in a medically underserved area.[20,21]

Wolinsky faults the model's low predictability power on the use of "static conceptualizations of dynamic causal processes."[22] In his longitudinal study of National Health Interview Survey data, the coefficients of illness-need variables were highly unstable over time. Mechanic suggests that imprecise specification of independent variables, such as measures of insurance coverage, and physician ratios, which are often based on large geographical areas, may contribute to a weak causal relationship between enabling variables and utilization outcomes.[23] With these limitations in mind, I modified the Behavioral model, in part, to include measures of residential instability; as such, it became the framework for conducting multivariate analyses.

SAMPLING

The research is based on data from a longitudinal study of mothers on welfare in New York City, who were first interviewed in 1988 (Time 1), and again beginning in 1992 through 1993 (Time 2). The first wave of interviews included two samples (see Figure 4.1). One sample comprised heads of households from 700 families, drawn randomly from the population of families requesting shelter at city-operated emergency assistance units (EAUs). EAUs are the point of intake for homeless families into the city's family shelter system (see Appendix A for a description). The second sample, a housed comparison group of 519 families selected via multi-stage cluster sampling, was interviewed at city welfare offices, called income maintenance centers (IMCs), during scheduled welfare re-certification appointments.

Household heads were eligible for the Time 1 study if they were receiving public assistance (or had been removed from public assistance rolls in the past six months); had not been in shelter within the past month; and met New York's definition of a family: one or more parents with at least one child, or a pregnant woman. The studies on homeless families by Knickman, Shinn and Weitzman that are referred to in the first three chapters are based on this Time 1 sample.

Figure 4.1
Time 1 and Time 2 Samples

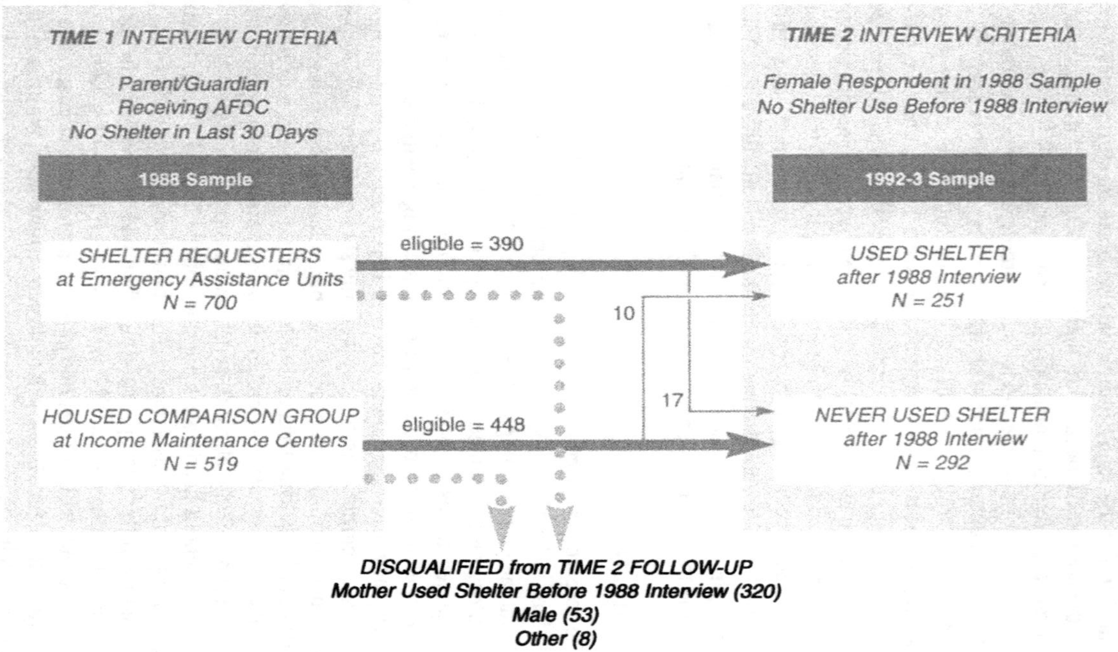

The second wave of the study excluded two major groups of respondents from the Time 1 study, namely, male households and those who had used shelter before the 1988 interview. Specifically, only women who met the public assistance criteria, who had children in their care or were pregnant at Time 1, and who had not used shelter more than one week prior to their initial interview were included in the Time 2 follow-up study. We used self-reports and administrative records to verify the latter. The final sample size of eligible respondents for the follow up study was 838 families.

RESPONSE RATES

Five years after the initial Time 1 study, the research team located 80 percent and re-interviewed 70 percent of the sample; this included 266, or 70 percent, of eligible mothers requesting shelter (excluding nine deceased respondents, confirmed by death certificates) and 298, or 69 percent, of the eligible comparison mothers (excluding ten deceased respondents). Interviewed respondents, overall, were highly representative of the total sample of eligible respondents, with few significant differences (see Appendix B for a comparison of mothers on a variety of characteristics at Time 1).

Some of the Time 2 respondents (n=21) declined to complete the full protocol and completed a short version in person or by phone or mail instead. We excluded these respondents from the analyses because their interviews were significantly incomplete. Because six respondents, two of whom were shelter-requesters, gave information during the Time 2 interview that led us to discover they had used shelter prior to their 1988 interview, we deleted their interviews from the sample. Thus, the full sample, on which the analyses are based, included data from 543 respondents' interviews, completed by 251 mothers who used shelter ("ever-sheltered") and 292 mothers who never used shelter ("never-sheltered").

As depicted in Figure 4.1, 17 of the mothers we classified as never-sheltered in the follow up study were actually interviewed at an EAU in 1988 as requesting shelter, but subsequently never used shelter. Ten of the mothers we classified as ever-sheltered were originally part of the housed comparison group, but used shelter sometime after their 1988 interview. We made the latter reclassification because this group used shelter and met the criterion of having no episode of shelter before Time 1.

For the follow-up study, we included children as respondents. Interviewers requested mothers to report health information on their children, for as many as one from each of four age groups (birth-2, 3-6, 7-10, and 11-17). The child in a given age group with the most recent birthday at the time of the interview was selected as a respondent, among children ages three and older. The child's mother or guardian provided all of the health-related data.

We did not collect health reports on children living outside of a mother's or guardian's household. Among children whom the mother identified as being other than her own, those 6 years old and younger were eligible to be interviewed if they had been part of the family for at least half the child's life; those between ages 7 through 17 were eligible if they had been part of the family since at least the time of the mother's 1988 interview.

Among mothers with a full, completed protocol, 470 had at least one child in one of the four target age groups. We collected health reports from mothers on all 207 eligible children in the 11-17 age group; on all but one child in the 7-10 age group, for a total of 207 reports; on 100 percent of the 219 eligible children in the 3-6 age group; and on 132 infants, with three reports missing. Overall, there are health reports from mothers for 765 children.

LOCATING AND INTERVIEWING FAMILIES

We faced numerous challenges attempting to locate families with whom we had had no contact for at least four years. Because the Time 1 study was originally designed as a one-time survey, researchers had made no attempt to maintain contact with families after mothers were interviewed in 1988. Only after the principal investigators received an entirely new grant to follow-up on the families did researchers implement a systematic approach for locating mothers and families.

We developed a "batch" system, for which our staff focused resources over a two to three week period to find and interview about 50 families at a time. Every three to four weeks, we started a search for a new batch of families, constantly tracking the progress and status of the earlier batches. This process continued for about two years. To our surprise, persistence paid off in a dramatic way. We located 100 percent of the families in the first batch, but only half of the families who made up the last batch.

By far, the most valuable resource for address information was the public assistance database system maintained by the New York City Human Resources Administration (HRA), the city's welfare agency. Most of the families in our study were still receiving public assistance, which required them to keep their addresses current with HRA. While interviewers had asked respondents during their Time 1 interview to provide the name and address of someone who would be likely to know her whereabouts in the future, this information proved only marginally helpful.

For each batch of families, research staff initially mailed a series of two letters, one week apart from each other, in both English and Spanish, to introduce families to the study and offer incentive payments. Interviewers followed-up the letters with personal visits and telephone calls, when a phone number was available. Neighbors, former neighbors, and contacts previously identified by respondents were queried if families could not be located by other means. Each time we obtained a new address, usually from HRA, we generated a new series of letters and visits.

Interviewers completed the surveys at a family's residence or at the research project office, based on the family's choice. Interviews were conducted in a single session, lasting up to three hours for mothers. We paid mothers $35 for their participation, plus a $15 transportation fee if they came to the research project offices at New York University. Respondents were interviewed in English or Spanish, at their preference. Interviewers, like respondents, were predominantly African-American and Latina, and several were fully bilingual. Interviewers participated in a training program of approximately 100 hours and received ongoing supervision.

DATA SOURCES

The analyses are based primarily on self-reported data collected during the Time 2 study period, from April, 1992 to December, 1993, and from the 1988 Time 1 survey. We asked mothers to provide demographic and family composition data, and to report on their shelter and/or housing histories; their history, if any, with substance abuse; and their use of welfare and social services since their Time 1 interview.

Mothers also reported on their family's health problems and use of health and mental health services for the twelve months prior to their Time 2 interview.

The Time 1 survey provided baseline data on mothers' housing and welfare histories, and their experiences with substance abuse and mental health problems. Baseline health-related data came from two sources. One was the self-reported data on mothers' health problems for the year preceding the 1988 interview. In addition, Medicaid records obtained from the New York State Department of Social Services provided health care utilization data for a sub-sample of 386 mothers during fiscal year 1986-87.

When interviewers began reporting from the field that a family member told them a respondent had died, we developed a process for requesting death statistics. Each time we received matching death information on a respondent from the National Death Index, a division of the U.S. Department of Health and Human Services, we requested and received a copy of a death certificate from the vital statistics department of the locality in which the respondent died (mainly New York City, but also Puerto Rico, Georgia and South Carolina). Mortality data on mothers eligible for the Time 2 study appear in Chapter 5 to supplement the discussion on health status.

Using hospital data published by the American Hospital Association,[24] we matched hospital zip codes with the zip code associated with the respondent's address (or place lived longest in the last year) to measure whether a hospital was located in a respondent's neighborhood.

DEVELOPMENT OF ANALYTICAL MODELS

We developed analytical models to examine the relationship between residential instability and health care use, controlling for other independent variables. We adapted measures of outpatient health care use from those used in the National Health Interview Survey.[25] Interviewers asked each mother about herself and each child, whether there was a place that they usually go when they "are sick or need advice about health matters," and what kind of place it was. We asked this question to elicit where each family member goes on a regular basis for medical care.

We also asked mothers how many times in the past 12 months that they and each of their children visited "a medical doctor or nurse, or someone working for a doctor, or [went] to a clinic, emergency room or a health department clinic" (excluding doctors seen during a hospital stay). While the source of care variable measures more explicitly where families go when they are sick, the variable for total visits is more implicit about the purpose of medical visits. Thus, the number of medical care visits reported may include sick or preventive care, or even a visit to an emergency department for illness or injury requiring urgent care. As described, the dependent variables measure, most generally, utilization of outpatient medical care, for which the terms "health care" and "medical care" are used interchangeably.

We developed one "template" model of independent variables for analyzing mothers' and children's utilization patterns. The template model, based on the health behavioral model and hypotheses, is represented by the following function:

Utilization = f(Predisposing (with Residential Instability) + Enabling + Need)

From this template are three models, one for each type of utilization by mothers, and one for each type of utilization by children.

The first type of model is the multinomial logistic regression (MLR) model (see Appendix C for a description) for analyzing regular source of care patterns. Among the four categories of the dependent variable for sources of care, Doctor/HMO is the base category from which all other categories are compared. This category does not necessarily represent higher quality medical care. Rather, it represents private sources of care, a distinction made by the National Health Interview Survey, in contrast to "clinic" care providers.[26] Clinic care includes public and/or hospital-based sources of care, such as hospital outpatient clinics (namely inner-city teaching hospitals), emergency departments and community clinics. Baxter and Mechanic refer to these as the "core safety net institutions."[27] Throughout the rest of the text, "mainstream" providers refer to private physicians, clinics and HMOs, and "safety net" providers refer to the public or hospital-based sources of care named above. The choice of a base category does not influence the overall results of a model. It does, however, reflect differences in any particular independent variable's association with one source of care *relative* to another source of care.

The second type of model is a logistic regression model with a dependent variable that measures whether or not any medical visits were made in the last twelve months (preceding the Time 2 interview). The third type is a linear regression model for examining the total volume of visits made in the last year.

RESIDENTIAL INSTABILITY FACTORS

The research variables of principle interest, namely measures of residential instability, include having ever used shelter and the degree of residential mobility before and after Time 1. These measures, listed below, refer to time frames that *preceded* the twelve months prior to a family's Time 2 interview, the period for which health care utilization was measured. For this reason, they are characterized as predisposing variables.

Shelter use, or shelter status, refers to whether a family, specifically a mother, ever stayed in shelter, regardless of the length of stay. For the purposes of this study, any mother or child of a mother in the sample who stayed in shelter after her 1988 interview is labeled "ever-sheltered" (even though a child of an ever-sheltered mother may have been born after the mother left shelter); all others are labeled "never-sheltered."

Residential mobility refers only to the number of *non-shelter* places of residence for a given time period. The following define measures of mobility:

Pre-Time 1 Mobility: Having lived in four or more places during a period of three years prior to the Time 1 interview (base is one to three places).

Post-Time 1 Mobility: Having lived in two or more places in the period between the Time 1 interview and one year before the follow up (Time 2) interview (base is one place).

These categorical variables were created from two originally continuous variables. Neither of the mobility variables has a normal distribution because so many families lived in only one place in the three to four year period after their first interview, and two or fewer places in the three years preceding the Time 1 interview. The extreme range in values made categorical variables an appropriate measure of mobility.

The process of dichotomizing these variables was an exploratory one to determine how much mobility seemed to make a difference. With no standard definitions of residential mobility to guide the analyses, the definitions used in these analyses represent thresholds at which a level of mobility is related to any of the utilization outcomes in bivariate analyses. For example, only at the threshold of four or more places is pre-Time 1 mobility related to utilization, specifically regular source of care patterns. Only 12 percent (n=65) of mothers experienced this high level of pre-Time 1 mobility; of those who did, 85 percent used shelter. This threshold, itself, suggests that only extreme levels of pre-Time 1 mobility, experienced mostly by shelter users, is related to current health care utilization.

The threshold of significance for Post-Time 1 mobility was much lower. In this case, mobility refers to living in more than one place, versus living in only one place between the Time 1 interview and one year before the Time 2 interview. This measure excludes the number of shelters families lived in during this period.

For the twelve months preceding Time 2, mobility was very low for both groups; less than 20 percent lived in more than one place in the last year. The analyses examined whether current residential stability was related to current utilization outcomes. Current stability is defined as having lived in one's own apartment independently (not doubled-up) for at least one year. Since measures of residential instability include mobility factors and shelter (a lack of housing independence), it is appropriate for current stability to include a combination of mobility (one place in the last year) and independence (one's own place). Current residential stability is an enabling factor because it refers to the same period—the twelve months prior to the Time 2 interview—as that used to measure health care use.

CONTROL VARIABLES

The model also contains a number of control variables, based on their theoretical significance regarding utilization patterns, as described in previous chapters. The inclusion of control variables was consistent, but not identical, across mothers' and children's models. While "family" variables, such as (mothers') welfare and employment status are identical in children's and mothers' models, individual variables such as age and health status are unique to the family member.

Language is an exception; the mother's language preference is used for her children as well. A variable concerning pregnancy in the last year is included in mothers' models only. And while most "enabling" factors are considered family variables, one exception is not having a regular source of care, which is measured for each family member. It is, in fact, included in the categories of the dependent variable for regular source of care, but it is also a control variable in the models for visit outcomes, based on other empirical research.[28]

The inclusion or exclusion of other control variables was based primarily on correlation analyses. For example, language preference rather than race/ethnicity was included in the models, with the former serving as a proxy for acculturation with English-speaking communities and institutions.[29] Race/ethnicity was excluded because it was highly correlated with language and correlated less strongly with the dependent variables. Of those with a preference for Spanish (27% of the sample), 58 percent were Puerto Rican and 41 percent were of other Hispanic descent. At the same time, only 42 percent of all Puerto Ricans preferred being interviewed in Spanish, while 80 percent of those of other Hispanic origin (who make up only 13 percent of the sample) preferred Spanish. Thus, while Spanish-speakers reflect Puerto Rican and other Hispanic families almost exclusively, English-speakers reflect a mix of black, Puerto Rican and other Hispanic families.

In addition, the total number of chronic health problems correlated more strongly with health care use than did health status. With the two measures highly correlated, only the former was included in the models.

The models include other predisposing factors, such as (the mother) having grown up with a parent on welfare, which is referred to as childhood poverty, and being pregnant or a new mother at Time 1. Both are strong predictors of shelter use.[30] Additionally, enabling factors, such as welfare status and trouble affording medical care were included in the models. Andersen and Newman did not specifically include these as enabling factors in their Behavioral model, but for this sample, initially selected, in part, based on being welfare-dependent, they serve as proxies of income, a factor which is included in the Behavioral Model.[31]

Variables such as educational level and marital status, which are included in the Behavioral model,[32] and used in general population studies of health care utilization, are excluded from the models. In earlier analyses, they were not associated with utilization outcomes, as is often the case in studies of low-income or welfare families.[33]

As discussed earlier in the literature review, factors related to mothers' psycho-social status are largely unrelated to health care utilization in studies of poor mothers. In preliminary analyses of this study, the variable for a mother's previous mental hospitalization (1.8% of sample) and a mother's previous jail stay (3.9% of sample) were associated with children having no medical visits in the previous year. Because so few mothers had these experiences, these factors produced extremely large standard errors, and different results for other factors when excluded. For these reasons, they were excluded from the multivariate analyses. While a relatively higher percentage (10.7%) of mothers had a history of substance abuse treatment, there is little evidence in the literature of a link with health care use. Since this factor was unrelated to the utilization outcomes examined, it was also excluded from the multivariate analyses.

Finally, while it is understood that mothers are making health care decisions on behalf of their children, the decisions they make for themselves may be based on different criteria or factors. Additionally, the direction of causality between mothers' and children's utilization is unclear. Therefore, neither was included as an independent variable in the other's model.

NOTES

1. Wolfe, B. L. (1980). Children's utilization of medical care. *Medical Care*, 18 (12), 1196-1207.
2. Andersen, R. M., & Newman, J. F. (1973). Societal and individual determinants of medical care utilization in the United States. *The Milbank Memorial Fund Quarterly*, 51(1), 95-121.
3. Andersen, R. M. (1995). Revisiting the behavioral model and access to medical care: Does it matter? *Journal of Health and Social Behavior*, 36, 1-10.
4. Andersen, R. M., & Newman, J. F. (1973), p. 107.
5. Litman, T. J. (1974). The family as a basic unit in health and medical care: A social behavioral overview. *Social Science Medicine*, 8, 495-519.
6. Andersen, R. M., & Newman, J. F. (1973).
7. Berkanovic, E., & Reeder, L. G. (1974). Can money buy the appropriate use of services? Some notes on the meaning of utilization data. *Journal of Health & Social Behavior*, 15 (June), 93-99.

8. Andersen, R. M., & Newman, J. F. (1973).

9. Wolinsky, F. D. (1978). Assessing the effects of predisposing, enabling and illness-morbidity characteristics on health service utilization. *Journal of Health and Social Behavior*, 19, 384-396.

10. Wolinsky, F. D. (1988). *The sociology of health: Principles, practitioners, and issues* (2nd ed.). Belmont, CA: Wadsworth Publishing Co.

11. Gelberg, L., Gallagher, T. C., Andersen, R. M., & Koegel, P. (1997). Competing priorities as a barrier to medical care among homeless adults in Los Angeles. *American Journal of Public Health*, 87 (2), 217-220.

12. Aday, L. A. (1993). Indicators and predictors of health services utilization. In S. J. Williams, & P. R. Torrens (Eds.), *Introduction to Health Services* (4th ed., pp. 46-70). Albany, NY: Delmar Publishing, Inc.

13. Kleinman, J. C., Gold, M., & Makuc, D. (1981). Use of ambulatory medical care by the poor: Another look at equity. *Medical Care*, 19 (10), 1011-1029.

14. Wolinsky, F. D. (1988).

15. Mechanic, D. (1979). Correlates of physician utilization: Why do major multivariate studies of physician utilization find trivial psychosocial and organizational effects? *Journal of Health and Social Behavior*, 20, 387-396.

16. Ibid.

17. Mechanic, D. (1989). Medical sociology: Some tensions among theory, method, and substance. *Journal of Health and Social Behavior*, 30, 147-160.

18. Wolinsky, F. D. (1978).

19. Wolinsky, F. D. (1982). Assessing the effects of the physical, psychological, and social dimensions of health on the use of health services. *The Sociological Quarterly*, 23, 191-206.

20. Wolinsky, F. D. (1978).

21. Mechanic, D. (1979).

22. Wolinsky, F. D. (1981). The problems for academic and entrepreneurial research in the use of health services. *The Sociological Quarterly*, 22, p. 221.

23. Mechanic, D. (1979).

24. American Hospital Association. (1994). *Guide to the Health Care Field.* Chicago, IL: Author.

25. National Center for Health Statistics. (1994). *National Health Interview Survey 1992*, Washington, DC: US Government Printing Office.

26. Bloom, B. (1995). Health insurance and medical care: Health of our nation's children, United States, 1988. *Advance data from vital and health*

statistics, (series 16, No. 19). Washington, DC: National Center for Health Statistics, p. 4.

27. Baxter, R. J., & Mechanic, R. E. (1997). The status of local health care safety nets. *Health Affairs*, 16 (4), p. 9.

28. Kuder, J. M., & Levitz, G. S. (1989). Visits to the physician: An evaluation of the usual-source effect. In G. H. DeFriese, III, T. C. Ricketts, & J. S. Stein (Eds.), *Methodological advances in health services research,* (pp. 193-209). Ann Arbor, MI: Health Administration Press.

29. Lewin-Epstein, N. (1991). Determinants of regular source of health care in Black, Mexican, Puerto Rican, and Non-Hispanic white populations. *Medical Care*, 29 (6), 543-557.

30. Knickman, J. R., Weitzman, B. C., Shinn M., & Marcus, E. H. (1989). *A study of homeless families in New York City: Characteristics and comparisons with other public assistance families* (Final Report: Volume 2). New York: New York University, Robert F. Wagner Graduate School of Public Service, Health Research Program.

31. Andersen, R. M., & Newman, J. F. (1973).

32. Andersen, R. M., Aday, L. A., & Chen, M. S. (1986). Health status and health care utilization. *Health Affairs*, 5 (1), 154-169.

33. Lewin-Epstein, N. (1991).

CHAPTER 5

Comparisons of Poor New York City Families by Shelter Use

For most sheltered families, homelessness is not a way of life but a bumpy path to stable, subsidized housing.[1] A period of residential instability often precedes a family's request for shelter, marked by a combination of living "doubled-up" and moving about among family and friends. For many, instability stems from a lack of household independence—never having had one's own apartment. For others, independence was interrupted by a fire, eviction or some other calamity. The statistics below illustrate the progress that most homeless families make, over time, towards achieving residential stability.

RESIDENTIAL INSTABILITY AND OTHER PREDISPOSING FACTORS

At the time they were first interviewed in 1988, three times as many ever-sheltered mothers reported they had *never* had their own apartment compared to never-sheltered mothers (Table 5.1). On average, ever-sheltered families experienced much more mobility than never-sheltered families in the three years prior to Time 1 (2.8 v. 1.4 places). By the time they were re-interviewed, 79 percent of ever-sheltered families were living in their own place. More than half—60 percent—had achieved residential stability: living in their own apartment or single room occupancy (SRO) for one year or longer. Almost three-quarters—72 percent—spent the longest part of the last year in their own apartment. At Time 2, ever-sheltered families had lived in their current place for two years, on average.

Table 5.1: Selected Residential Factors

	Ever-sheltered (N=251)	Never-sheltered (N=292)
Pre-Time 1 Period		
Never had Own Apartment before Time 1	43%	14%**
Pre-Time 1 Mobility mean (s.d.) *(№. Places Lived 3 Years before Time 1)*	2.8 (2.6)	1.4 (1.1)**
At Follow-up Interview		
Place Currently Living		
Own Apartment/SRO	79%	92%**
With Parents/Other Family/ Friend	14%	8%
Shelter/Other Place	7%	<1%
Achieved Residential Stability *(In own apt. or SRO for at least 1 year)*	60%	80%**
Years in Current Place mean (s.d.)	2.1 (1.5)	7.9 (6.7)**
Median Years in Current Place	2.1	6.9
Post-Time 1 Mobility mean (s.d.) *(№. Places Lived b/w Time 1 & 1 Year before Time 2)*	2.6 (3.9)	1.7 (1.3)**
Year Prior to Follow-up		
Place stayed longest		
Own Apartment/SRO	72%	92%**
With Parents/Other Family/ Friend	15%	8%
Shelter/Other Place	13%	<1%
Last Year Mobility mean (s.d.) *(№. Places Lived)*	1.2 (0.5)	1.2 (0.4)

*P < .05; ** P < .01

While ever-sheltered families made considerable progress in achieving residential stability, most never-sheltered families had stayed put in their own place through the entire study period, averaging eight years in their current place. This phenomenon illustrates the power of a tight, subsidized housing market in New York City. Once a family finds a relatively affordable place, it is unlikely to move, despite even lousy housing conditions, because so little else is available. Formerly homeless families, having waited in the shelter system queue for subsidized housing, typically for a year or more, are tapping into this same supply, for which vacancies are rare and waiting lists are long.

Currently, more than 215,000 people in New York City are in the queue for receiving rent subsidies, for which homeless families receive highest priority.[2] Few can afford to give up what they waited so long to obtain, which may explain why ever-sheltered families, 94 percent of whom were no longer homeless at Time 2, had essentially no mobility in the 12 months prior to their Time 2 interview. Only a minority of ever-sheltered families were still struggling with residential instability at Time 2, with 13 percent spending the longest portion of the previous 12 months, in a shelter, in a public place or institution, such as a prison or mental hospital, or in some other setting.

DEMOGRAPHIC AND SOCIAL STRUCTURE FACTORS

Overall, the demographic profile of ever- and never-sheltered families in New York City is consistent with those made from studies of homeless and housed families in other major U.S. urban areas.[3,4] As with their housing histories, ever-sheltered families look quite different than other poor families on predisposing factors such as age and race (Table 5.2).

Because age is highly related to health, family size and other "life cycle" factors,[5] we could expect age to account for statistical differences between ever-sheltered and never-sheltered families on a number of characteristics. Ever-sheltered mothers are significantly younger, on average, than never-sheltered mothers (32 v. 39). Likewise, ever-sheltered children are also younger, on average (7. v. 9). To help determine whether shelter status remained statistically associated with a factor after controlling for age, a number of factors were regressed onto mothers' age and shelter status, with the results described in the text, where appropriate. For example, even after controlling for age, shelter status remains highly associated with residential factors, although age is also associated with never having had one's own apartment, and the amount of time lived in the current place.

Table 5.2: Predisposing Characteristics at Follow-Up

	Ever-sheltered (N=251)	Never-sheltered (N=292)
Age mean, (std. dev.)		
Mothers' Age	32 (6.8)	39 (10.1)**
Children's Age	7 (4.5)	9 (4.6)**
Mothers' Race/Ethnicity		
Black	58%	35%**
Puerto Rican	31%	41%
Other Hispanic	7%	19%
Other	4%	5%
Language Preference		
Spanish	13%	38%**
English	87%	62%
Marital Status		
Single/Never Married	56%	37%**
Married	16%	14%
Divorced, Separated, Other	28%	49%
Childhood Poverty *(Mother had a Parent on Welfare When Growing Up)*	54%	28%**
New Mother or Pregnant at Time 1 (1988)	54%	17%**
Family Size mean, (std. dev.) *(Mean No. Children <18 living w/ Mother)*	2 (1.7)	2 (1.3)
Education		
High School Graduate/GED	45%	44%

*P < .05; ** P < .01

Regardless of shelter status, poor families in New York City are overwhelmingly non-white. However, ever-sheltered families are more likely to be black (58% v. 35%), than either Puerto Rican (31% v. 41%) or of other Hispanic descent (7% v. 19%). Language preferences mirror ethnic differences by shelter status, with never-sheltered mothers much more likely to prefer speaking Spanish.

Literature on family poverty has noted welfare's disincentives toward marriage.[6] Not surprisingly, marriage rates for sampled mothers are much lower than those found in the general population, with rates of 14 and 16 percent, respectively, for ever-sheltered and never-sheltered mothers. Nationally, marriage rates hover around 45 percent for black women and 76 percent for white women between ages 25 to 44.[7] Rates for sampled mothers are also much lower than those reported by Woods and Valdez[8] for homeless (47%) and housed (38%) mothers, and those reported by Winkleby and Boyce[9] for homeless mothers (41%). Ever-sheltered mothers were more likely to report having never married, and never-sheltered mothers were more likely to report being divorced or separated, characteristics which appear to be related to the race and age differences of the samples, since age, but not shelter use, was statistically associated with marriage status.

In the Time 1 study, Shinn, Knickman, and Weitzman found that childhood poverty, that is, growing up with at least one parent on welfare, was a predictor of family homelessness.[10] In the Time 2 sample, childhood poverty remains much more common among ever-sheltered (54%) than never-sheltered mothers (28%). Being a new mother or pregnant also predicted family shelter use at Time 1.[11] For the Time 2 sample, more than half—54 percent—of ever-sheltered mothers had been pregnant or had become a new mother at the time of their 1988 interview. Despite their age and other differences, ever-sheltered and never-sheltered families are similar in family size and educational attainment. Among both groups, family size averages two children under 18 years of age in the mother's custody. Less than half of the mothers have a high school diploma or General Equivalency Diploma (GED).

FAMILY AND COMMUNITY ENABLING FACTORS

Only a minority of mothers were currently employed at Time 2 (Table 5.3), with ever-sheltered mothers being significantly less so than never-sheltered mothers (6% v. 14%). Age did not explain this difference. About one-third of mothers (35%, ever-sheltered v. 30%, never-sheltered) had worked 20 hours per week, or more, at some point after their 1988 interview. The majority of mothers were still on public assistance approximately five years after their initial interview (86%, ever-sheltered v. 71%, never-sheltered). Older mothers are more likely to have had children turn 18 years old, or "age out," disqualifying the mother from public assistance eligibility. In a simple regression analysis with two independent variables, age was highly related to being off public assistance, while shelter use was not.

Table 5.3: Family & Community Enabling Factors at Follow-up

	Ever-sheltered (N=251)	Never-sheltered (N=292)
Employment/Public Assistance		
Currently Employed	6%	14%**
Ever Worked 20 hrs/wk after Time 1	35%	30%
Currently on Public Assistance (PA)	86%	71%**
PA Case Closed Twice or More after Time 1	20%	9%**
Other Family Factors		
Can't Afford Medical Care	25%	20%
Mother Incarcerated after Time 1	8%	1%**
Community Enabling Factors		
Hospital in Family's Neighborhood	37%	25%**

*P < .05; ** P < .01

Among those on public assistance at Time 2, ever-sheltered mothers, however, were significantly more likely to have had multiple welfare-case closings since 1988 (20% v. 9%), suggesting that homelessness and disruptions in welfare benefits may be related. When asked a series of questions about "economic stressors," one-quarter of ever-sheltered and one-fifth of never-sheltered mothers reported that often or very often they did not have enough money to afford the medical care their family should have. Public assistance does not correlate with this response, suggesting that even with Medicaid coverage as a welfare benefit, cost can be a barrier to health care access, as discussed in Chapter 2.

The key community enabling variable included in the model was the presence of a neighborhood hospital. Ever-sheltered families were more likely to be living in a neighborhood with a hospital (37% v.

25%), as defined by matching zip codes, but there is no indication that homelessness or housing opportunities are related to this statistic or other neighborhood characteristics. In fact, both ever-sheltered and never-sheltered families live in some of New York City's poorest neighborhoods, which tend to have high concentrations of welfare families. Ever-sheltered families relocated into poor neighborhoods, but not necessarily the poorest; nor did their addresses cluster into particular neighborhoods.

Family Health Status

The health statistics from this study lend further evidence that the chronic health problems of poor families are far more attributable to poverty than to homelessness (Table 5.4). When controlling for age, shelter status is unrelated to mothers' and children's health. Nor is shelter use related to chronic or functionally limiting health problems or being pregnant in the last year, once age is controlled for. Both ever-sheltered and never-sheltered mothers have higher rates of fair or poor health status, and health problems that limit daily functioning, compared to a national, representative sample of women surveyed in the 1992 National Health Interview Survey (NHIS).[12] While 34 percent of ever-sheltered and 47 percent of never-sheltered mothers reported being in fair or poor health, the same was true for only 8 percent of women between ages 25 and 44 (18% for those between 45 and 64) surveyed by NHIS. Children's rates of fair/poor health status varied little by shelter status (16% v. 18%) across all age groups. These rates are very similar to those that Wood and Valdez found for sheltered (17%) and housed (13%) children, as reported by their mothers.[13]

According to their self-reports, 75 percent of mothers and half of their children, regardless of shelter status, suffer from one or more chronic health conditions. Among the most commonly reported for mothers are asthma, back problems, stomach problems, and anemia. Excluding back problems, these same conditions were the most common ones facing children as well; ear infections were another. Rates are nearly identical for ever-sheltered and never-sheltered children. These findings may reflect the fact that living conditions in family shelters have improved over time, while housing and environmental conditions remain unhealthy for many poor families residing in New York City.

Table 5.4: Selected Health Characteristics for the Last Year

	Ever-sheltered Mothers, N=251 Children, N=385	Never-sheltered Mothers, N=292 Children, N=380
Fair/Poor Health Status		
Mothers	34%	47%**
Children	14%	18%
At least 1 Chronic Health Problem		
Mothers	75%	77%
Children	50%	52%
Selected Chronic and Other Conditions		
Stomach problems		
Mothers	16%	22%
Children	8%	7%
Anemia		
Mothers	26%	25%
Children	10%	11%
Asthma		
Mothers	19%	22%
Children	21%	21%
Ear Infections		
Children	17%	21%
Back Problems		
Mothers	27%	37%*
Mother Pregnant	25%	10%**
Impact of Health Problems		
Health Problem(s) Limits Mother's Daily Functioning, at Time 2	18%	29%**
Health Problem(s) Limited Mother's Daily Functioning, at Time 1	13%	23%*

*P < .05; ** P < .01

Health problems that limit daily functioning are also more common among the sampled mothers than the general population of women. Only 14 percent of an NHIS sample of women ages 25 to 44 (21% for women ages 45 to 64) reported having a health problem that limits daily functioning,[14] compared to 18 percent and 29 percent of ever-sheltered and never-sheltered women, respectively. Both groups of mothers had similar increases in these rates (5% and 6%, respectively) between their first and second interviews.

Children's Birth Outcomes

On one measure of health, ever-sheltered families look decidedly different. As shown in Table 5.5, a higher percentage of children from ever-sheltered families (14%) were born prematurely, compared to children of never-sheltered families (9%), according to mothers' reports.

Table 5.5: Birth Outcomes Reported By Mothers at Follow-up[a]

Children's Birth Outcomes	Ever-sheltered (N=381)	Never-sheltered (N=374)
Premature Birth		
All Age Groups[b]	14%	9%*
11-17 years old	8%	7%
7-10	15%	11%
3-6	15%	7%
0-2	17%	10%
Low Birth-weight		
< 5.5 lbs.		
All Age Groups[b]	19%	11%**
11-17 years old	20%	12%
7-10	17%	11%
3-6	19%	11%
0-2	22%	8%*
Mean Birth-weight		
lbs., mean (s.d)		
All Age Groups[b]	6.7 (1.5)	7.1 (1.4)**
11-17 years old	6.8 (1.4)	7.1 (1.4)
7-10	6.6 (1.5)	7.2 (1.6)**
3-6	6.6 (1.4)	7.1 (1.4)*
0-2	6.8 (1.7)	7.3 (1.3)

[a] Mothers did not report on children who were not biologically related to them.

[b] Sample sizes for age groups: 11-17: N_s=76, N_{ns}=129; 7-10: N_s=101, N_{ns}=104; 3-6: N_s=124, N_{ns}=93; 0-2: N_s=80, N_{ns}=48, where N_s refers to Ever-Sheltered samples and N_{ns} refers to Never-Sheltered samples.

*P < .05; ** P < .01

While these data cannot be corroborated by medical data, they are congruent with medically-based outcomes reported in the literature.[15,16] The numbers are too small to show a statistically significant difference by age sub-group, but the pattern is consistent, except for 11 to 17 year olds. Their outcomes look much better on premature birth. Notably, children in this age group were born at least five years before their mother entered shelter.

A significantly higher portion of ever-sheltered children (19% v. 11%) were born with low birth weight, defined as below 2500 grams (approximately 5.5 lbs.). In this case, differences hold up across all age groups, including 11 to 17 year olds, and 0 to 2 year olds, who were born after most mothers had left shelter. In New York City, the rate of low birth weight was 9.7 percent of live births in 1991.[17]

The average birth weight is also significantly lower for ever-sheltered than never-sheltered children (6.7 lbs. v. 7.1 lbs.). The pattern is almost constant across age groups, but differences are statistically significant only for 7 to 10 year olds and 3 to 6 year olds. Among homeless families, the former were born at the peak of their mother's residential instability before entering shelter. The latter were born at the height of their mother's stay in shelter. The lack of significance for the oldest and youngest age groups may be a result of their smaller sub-group sample sizes. Shelter status remains a significant predictor of each of these three outcomes for combined age groups, even after controlling for ethnicity and other factors associated with birth outcomes.

AIDS and Mortality

AIDS, a leading cause of death among minority women in New York City, ages 25 to 44,[18] was the leading cause of death of mothers eligible for the Time 2 follow up study. Of the 19 women who died after their first interview, five of nine (56%) ever-sheltered mothers and four of ten (40%) never-sheltered mothers died of AIDS, as confirmed by their death certificate. Seven of eight respondents who said they were HIV positive or had AIDS were women who used shelter. The numbers are too small to draw conclusions about the relationship between family homelessness and AIDS. However, the fact remains that both ever-sheltered and never-sheltered mothers represent poor, minority women who are at high-risk for contracting the AIDS virus. Other causes of mortality also highlight the health and environmental risks facing poor, urban mothers. They included cancer (3 cases), asthma (2 cases), and individual cases of hypertension, diabetes, suicide, drug overdose, and burns from a household fire.

Health Status Summary

When ever-sheltered families are compared to never-sheltered families between four and five years after initially becoming homeless, their health status and rates of chronic health conditions appear rather similar. These findings do not dismiss homelessness as a contributing factor to acute illnesses or poor maternal and birth outcomes experienced during the course of living in emergency shelter. The birth outcomes presented above suggest that mothers who have experienced residential instability may be at risk for worse birth outcomes, not just during shelter use, but before and after as well. However, the data sets by age group are too small to make firm conclusions. These findings further highlight the need for research on the relationship between health and homelessness before and beyond the period of living in shelter.

Despite their higher percentages of premature birth and low birth weight, children from ever-sheltered families do not appear to suffer chronic health problems at levels higher than other children born into poverty, at least not four to five years after their mothers first became homeless. When ever-sheltered and never-sheltered families—both mothers and children—are compared to general populations, poverty's contribution to higher rates of chronic illness seems grimly clear.

HEALTH CARE HEALTH UTILIZATION

Regular Source of Primary Care

In contrast to the lack of differences found in rates of chronic health conditions, ever-sheltered and never-sheltered families show striking differences regarding where they seek health care. The majority of families have a regular source of care (Table 5.6), although ever-sheltered mothers are significantly more likely *not* to have a regular source of care, and mothers are more likely than their children not to have a regular source of care. Nationally, 12 percent of children under 18 years of age do not have a regular source of care.[19]

Table 5.6: Families' Regular Source of Care for the Last Year

	Ever-sheltered Mothers, N=251 Children, N=385	**Never-sheltered** Mothers, N=292 Children, N=380
Has No Regular Source of Care		
Mothers	12%	4%***
Children	5%	3%
With a Regular Source of Care	Mothers, N=221 Children, N=365	Mothers, N=272 Children, N=370
Emergency Department		
Mothers	12%	3%**
Children	10%	4%**
Community/PH Clinic		
Mothers	25%	11%**
Children	31%	15%**
Hospital Outpatient Dept		
Mothers	31%	27%
Children	25%	18%*
Private Physician/HMO		
Mothers	26%	56%**
Children	31%	60%**
Other		
Mothers	1%	<1%
Children	3%	2%

*P < .05; ** P < .01

Compared to their never-sheltered counterparts, ever-sheltered mothers have four times the rate of emergency department (ED) use as a regular source of care (12% v. 3%), and their children have more than twice the rate (10% v. 4%). By definition, an emergency department is not intended as a regular source of primary care. It is not an appropriate setting for the care of chronic illnesses or preventive care services. Therefore, it could be argued that using an ED for these kinds of primary care services is tantamount to not having a regular source of care. In fact, those who reported an ED as their regular source of care had more variation in where they went for their most recent visit than respondents reporting any other source of care. Forty percent of ED respondents had visited a place *other* than an ED on their last medical care visit. Only 11 percent of those who reported regularly using either a private physician/HMO or a hospital OPD had used a different source during their most recent visit.

Overall, of mothers who indicated having a regular source of care, about 85 percent had used that source of care most recently. The only group with more variation than ED users were those without a regular source of care. The main difference between the two is that those without a regular source of care are heavier users of community/public health clinics and lighter users of emergency departments. With the categories combined, three times as many ever-sheltered mothers (23% v. 8%) and twice as many ever-sheltered children (14% v. 7%) use an ED or have no regular source of care, compared to their never-sheltered counterparts. This new category of ED/No Regular Source of Care is used in the multivariate analyses.

Ever-sheltered families use community/public health (PH) clinics (neighborhood health clinics, Well Child Health stations and Department of Health clinics) at twice the rate of never-sheltered families. At the same time, reliance on a hospital outpatient department (OPD) as a regular source of care does not differ significantly by shelter status. Nearly one-third of all mothers rely on a hospital OPD as their regular source of care. Children are less dependent on a hospital OPD than their mothers, but ever-sheltered children rely on them significantly more than never-sheltered children.

Families' reliance on private physicians/HMOs differs enormously by shelter status. Age does not account for these differences. Never-sheltered mothers rely on private physicians/HMOs at more than twice the rate of ever-sheltered mothers (56% v. 26%). The differences are just as extreme for children, and appear even more so when compared to nationally representative survey statistics. Based on NHIS data, of those with a regular source of care, about 16 percent of children under age 18 use a source of care other than a private physician or HMO; the rate rises to 23 percent for the central city, and is highest, at almost 37 percent, for those with family annual incomes under $10,000.[20] Yet, of ever-sheltered children with a regular source of care, a whopping 69 percent use a source of care other than a private physician or HMO.

The same is true for 40 percent of never-sheltered children, which is more in line with national statistics on families living in poverty.

Mothers' Baseline Utilization

One explanation for differences in source of regular care by shelter status is that ever-sheltered mothers used health care differently even before they requested shelter. Although incomplete for the sample, Medicaid utilization data on 386 mothers from fiscal year 1986-87 suggest that differences, at least in emergency department use, may predate shelter use. Whereas 41 percent of ever-sheltered mothers had at least one visit to an emergency department during that year, only 27 percent of never-sheltered mothers did. With 79 percent of never-sheltered mothers and only 62 percent of ever-sheltered mothers represented, these data are themselves biased towards never-sheltered mothers. Attempts to find other factors associated with having baseline data showed that, in a logit analysis, only shelter status was a statistically significant factor.

Medical Visits

Two aspects of medical visit patterns were of research interest: having any visits, and the total number of visits in the twelve months before the Time 2 interview. The former reflects having any access, while the latter measures the level of overall utilization. Table 5.7 shows that neither measure differs significantly by shelter status for mothers or children. Because the standard deviations are quite high, medians are also presented. The median values also show that the volume of annual medical visits is similar for sheltered and never-sheltered families.

Compared to national statistics, both ever-sheltered and never-sheltered families are high users of outpatient medical care. Nationally, children (under 15) average 2.6 visits per year, and women between ages 25 and 44 average 3.2 visits (and 3.6 visits for women between ages 45 and 64).[21]

Table 5.7: Medical Visit Utilization in the Last Year

	Ever-sheltered Mothers, N=251 Children, N=385	**Never-sheltered** Mothers, N=292 Children, N=380
No Medical Visits		
Mothers	7%	7%
Children	8%	7%
Annual Medical Care Visits *mean (s.d.)*		
Mothers	8 (12)	9 (12)
Children	6 (9)	5 (6)
Annual Medical Care Visits *median*		
Mothers	4	5
Children	4	4

*P<.05; ** P<.01; *** P<.001

Non-Primary Care Utilization

As shown in Table 5.8, below, there was little difference in hospitalization rates by shelter status, for either mothers (18%, ever-sheltered v. 15%, never-sheltered, excluding childbirth) or children (8%, ever-sheltered v. 7%, never-sheltered) for the year preceding the Time 2 interview. However, these rates are *more than double* comparable rates in the general population (6% to 8%, women 18 to 64 years old; 3% to 4% for boys and girls under 18).[22] By contrast, mental hospitalization appears to be rare among both ever- and never-sheltered mothers, a finding supported by the literature.[23] Three percent of ever-sheltered and 1 percent of never-sheltered mothers reported a mental hospital admission after 1988.

The similarities end with substance abuse. About one-sixth of ever-sheltered mothers reported using rehabilitation (rehab) services for alcohol and/or drug abuse after being interviewed in 1988, compared to less than 6 percent for never-sheltered mothers. During the baseline Time 1 interviews, less than 5 percent of either group reported having *ever* used rehab services. These figures do not represent the prevalence of substance abuse nor the need for treatment, only an estimate of service use. Whether being part of the shelter system increased the likelihood of homeless mothers developing a substance abuse problem, or the likelihood of being identified for or pressured into treatment (e.g., concerning child custody), or both, are questions for future research, and beyond the scope of this study.

Table 5.8: Inpatient Care Utilization in the Last Year

	Ever-sheltered Mothers, N=251 Children, N=385	**Never-sheltered** Mothers, N=292 Children, N=380
Hospitalized (excluding birth)		
Mothers	18%	15%
Children	8%	7%
Mental Hospitalization		
Mother Hospitalized for Mental Health Problems after Time 1	3%	1%
Inpatient Rehab Stay		
Mother in Substance Abuse Rehab after Time 1	16%	6%**

*P < .05; ** P < .01

Summary of Health Care Utilization

The data presented suggest that ever-sheltered mothers are different from other poor mothers in where they seek primary health care. Based on a limited sample, they used emergency care more frequently than never-sheltered mothers did, during the year that preceded their first entry into shelter. Unknown is whether this higher utilization was a result of a greater need for urgent or emergency medical attention, or whether it reflects a greater reliance on the emergency department as a regular source of primary health care.

The Time 2 data show that ever-sheltered families continued to have a relatively high degree of ED use after they left shelter and, for the most part, had found permanent housing. Despite significant differences in source of care patterns, ever-sheltered and never-sheltered families obtained similar amounts of health care during the year preceding their Time 2 interview.

NOTES

1. Shinn M., Weitzman B. C., Stojanovic, D., Knickman J.R., Jimenez L., Duchon L., James S., Krantz D. (1998). Predictors of homelessness from shelter request to housing stability among families in New York City. *American Journal of Public Health*, 8 (12), in press.

2. Kennedy, R. (1998, March 4). Availability of rent aid is reduced. *The New York Times*, pp. B1, B6.

3. Bassuk, E. L., Buckner, J. C., Weinreb, L. F., Browne, A., Bassuk, S. S., Dawson, R., Perloff, J. N. (1997). Homelessness in female-headed families: Childhood and adult risk and protective factors. *American Journal of Public Health*, 87 (2), 241-248.

4. Wood, D., & Valdez, R. B. (1991). Barriers to medical care for homeless families compared with housed poor families. *American Journal of Diseases of Children*, 145 (10), 1109-1115.

5. Litman, T. J. (1974). The family as a basic unit in health and medical care: A social behavioral overview. *Social Science Medicine*, 8, 495-519.

6. Mead, L. M. (1992). *The New Politics of Poverty*. New York: Basic Books.

7. Wilson, W. J. & Neckerman, K. M. (1986). Poverty and family structure: The widening gap between evidence and public policy issues. In S.H. Danziger and D. H. Weinberg (Eds.), *Fighting Poverty* (pp. 232-259). Cambridge, MA: Harvard University Press.

8. Wood, D., & Valdez, R. B. (1991).

9. Winkleby, M. A., & Boyce, W. T. (1994). Health-related risk factors of homeless families and single adults. *Journal of Community Health*, 19 (February), 7–23.

10. Shinn, M., Knickman, J. R., Weitzman, B.C. (1991). Social relationships and vulnerability to becoming homeless among families. *American Psychologist*, 46, 1190-1187.

11. Weitzman, B. C. (1989). Pregnancy and childbirth: Risk factors for homelessness? *Family Planning Perspectives*, 21 (4), 175-178.

12. National Center for Health Statistics. (1994). *National Health Interview Survey 1992*, Washington, DC: US Government Printing Office.

13. Wood, D., & Valdez, R. B. (1991).

14. National Center for Health Statistics. (1994).

15. Chavkin, W., Kristal, A., Seabron, C., & Guigli, P. E. (1987). Reproductive experiences of women living in hotels for the homeless in New York City. *New York State Journal of Medicine*, 87, 10-13.

16. Burg, M. A. (1994). Health problems of sheltered homeless women and their dependent children. *Health & Social Work,* 19 (2), 125-131.

17. United Hospital Fund (1994). *New York City Community Health Atlas.* New York: Author.

18. Office of Vital Statistics. (1992). *Summary of vital statistics 1989.* New York: Department of Health.

19. Bloom, B. (1995). Health insurance and medical care: Health of our nation's children, United States, 1988. *Advance data from vital and health statistics,* (series 16, No. 19). Washington, DC: National Center for Health Statistics.

20. Ibid.

21. National Center for Health Statistics. (1992). *National Ambulatory Medical Care Survey 1989*, (series 13, No. 110) Washington, DC: US Government Printing Office.

22. National Center for Health Statistics. (1994).

23. Shinn, M., & Weitzman, B. C. (1996). Homeless families are different. In J. Baumohl (Ed.), *Homelessness in America: A reference book* (pp. 109-122). New York: Oryx Press.

CHAPTER 6

Health Care Use among Poor Families in New York City

This chapter presents the results of the multivariate analyses conducted on the health care utilization models described in Chapter 4. Results are discussed for mothers' and children's models for the general analyses and for the sub-group analyses of ever-sheltered families.

REGULAR SOURCE OF CARE

Even after controlling for predisposing, enabling, and illness factors, shelter use and pre-Time 1 mobility are highly associated with regular source of care patterns (Tables 6.1 and 6.2). Families who ever used shelter have significantly increased relative risks for using safety net providers over private physicians/HMOs, compared to never-sheltered families. Recall from the last chapter that the category of emergency department (ED) as a regular source of care was combined with the category of reporting no regular source of care, to create the outcome ED/No Regular Source. Note that with these categories separated, the residential instability factors produced similar risk ratios for each outcome, but with larger standard errors, due to the smaller cell sizes.

Mothers who experienced a high degree of mobility prior to requesting shelter in 1988 have 4.5 times the relative risk of using an ED or having no regular source of care over using private physicians/HMOs, and three times the relative risk of using community/public health (PH) clinics. Shelter use is associated with a higher relative risk of using a hospital OPD as a regular source of care.

Table 6.1: Multivariate Model for Mothers' Regular Source of Care

Mothers (N=538)	Hospital OPD (n=159)	Community/PH Clinic (n=87)	ED/No Reg Source (n=78)
	RRR[a] (95% CI[b])	RRR (95% CI)	RRR (95% CI)
Predisposing Factors			
Mother's Age	1.0 (1.0, 1.0)	1.0 (1.0, 1.0)	1.0 (1.0, 1.1)
Prefers Speaking Spanish	0.9 (0.5, 1.6)	0.1 (0.0, 0.4)**	0.5 (0.2, 1.1)
Experienced Childhood Poverty	0.8 (0.5, 1.3)	2.1 (1.2, 3.9)*	1.0 (0.5, 1.9)
Pregnant/New Mother in 1988	1.1 (0.6, 1.9)	1.3 (0.7, 2.5)	3.1 (1.5, 6.1)**
Family Size	0.9 (0.8, 1.1)	1.1 (0.9, 1.3)	1.1 (0.9, 1.4)
Residential Instability			
Pre-Time 1 Mobility	2.2 (0.9, 5.2)	2.9 (1.2, 7.4)*	4.5 (1.8, 11.3)**
Ever Used Shelter	2.7 (1.6, 4.5)**	2.3 (1.2, 4.3)**	2.9 (1.4, 5.9)**
Post-Time 1 Mobility	0.9 (0.6, 1.4)	1.1 (0.6, 2.0)	1.2 (0.6, 2.3)
Family & Community Enabling Factors			
Residential Stability	0.8 (0.5, 1.4)	0.7 (0.4, 1.3)	0.4 (0.2, 0.7)**
Currently Employed	0.6 (0.3, 1.4)	0.6 (0.2, 1.7)	0.5 (0.2, 1.5)
Not on Public Assistance	1.5 (0.8, 2.9)	1.0 (0.4, 2.5)	2.5 (1.1, 5.7)*
Can't afford medical care	0.9 (0.5, 1.7)	1.4 (0.7, 2.8)	3.3 (1.6, 6.5)**
Hospital in Family's Neighborhood	1.0 (0.6, 1.6)	0.7 (0.4, 1.3)	0.8 (0.4, 1.5)
Illness/Need Factors			
Nº. of Chronic Health Problems	1.1 (1.0, 1.3)*	0.9 (0.8, 1.1)	0.8 (0.7, 1.0)*
Pregnant in Last Year	1.2 (0.6, 2.4)	0.9 (0.4, 1.8)	1.6 (0.7, 3.5)

[a]RRR: Relative Risk Ratio; comparison is to a Private Doctor/HMO (n=214); [b]CI: confidence interval
*P < .05; **P < .01

Table 6.2: Multivariate Model for Children's Regular Source of Care

Children (N=748)	Hospital OPD (n=161)	Community/ PH Clinic (n=169)	ED/No Reg Source (n=80)
	RRR[a] (95% CI[b])	RRR (95% CI)	RRR (95% CI)
Predisposing Factors			
Child's Age	1.0 (0.9, 1.0)	1.0 (1.0, 1.1)	1.0 (0.9, 1.1)
Mother Prefers Speaking Spanish	0.5 (0.3, 0.9)*	0.1 (0.0, 0.2)**	0.6 (0.2, 1.3)
Mother Experienced Childhood Poverty	0.5 (0.3, 0.8)**	1.3 (0.9, 2.1)	0.7 (0.4, 1.3)
Mother Pregnant/New Mother in 1988	0.8 (0.5, 1.3)	1.3 (0.9, 2.1)	1.1 (0.6, 2.0)
Family Size	1.0 (0.8, 1.1)	1.0 (0.9, 1.2)	1.3 (1.1, 1.6)**
Residential Instability			
Pre-Time 1Mobility	1.4 (1.0, 1.9)	1.2 (0.9, 1.7)	2.0 (1.3, 2.9)**
Ever Used Shelter	2.2 (1.4, 3.4)**	2.4 (1.5, 3.8)**	2.6 (1.4, 5.1)**
Post-Time 1 Mobility	1.4 (0.9, 2.1)	1.4 (0.9, 2.2)	1.3 (0.8, 2.4)
Family & Community Enabling Factors			
Residential Stability	1.5 (0.9, 2.4)	1.2 (0.8, 1.9)	1.1 (0.6, 2.1)
Currently Employed	0.9 (0.3, 2.1)	0.4 (0.2, 0.9)*	0.6 (0.2, 1.8)
Not on Public Assistance	0.4 (0.2, 0.9)*	1.2 (0.6, 2.5)	2.0 (0.9, 4.8)
Can't afford medical care	1.0 (0.6, 1.7)	0.9 (0.5, 1.6)	5.3 (2.9, 9.7)**
Hospital in Family's Neighborhood	2.1 (1.4, 3.2)**	0.9 (0.5, 1.4)	2.1 (1.2, 3.6)*
Illness/Need Factors			
Nº. of Chronic Health Problems	1.1 (0.9, 1.3)	0.9 (0.8, 1.1)	0.6 (0.5, 0.8)**

[a]RRR: Relative Risk Ratio; comparison is to a Private Doctor/HMO (n=336); [b]CI: confidence interval
*P < .05; **P < .01

Table 6.1 also shows that current residential stability is a positive—or enabling—factor in reducing poor families' reliance on emergency departments or no regular source of care. However, a *history* of residential instability has as much or more influence on increasing families' relative risk of ED use or having no regular source of care as does current stability in reducing this risk. Although the ratios are not as large, children from ever-sheltered families also have an increased relative risk of using a hospital OPD, a community/PH clinic or an ED/No regular source of care, over a private doctor/HMO (Table 6.2). Pre-time 1 mobility also significantly increases children's relative risk of using an ED/No regular source of care (RRR=3.0), over a private doctor/HMO.

MEDICAL CARE VISITS

Neither factors of residential instability nor current residential stability were related to whether or not mothers or children made any medical care visits in the 12 months prior to the Time 2 interview (Table 6.3). Recall from Chapter 5 that only a small percentage of families went without any visits in the last year (8% for mothers, 4% for children).

In measuring the number of medical visits, outlier observations can bias results. The data were converted to natural logarithms to address this problem (which has the effect of eliminating observations with zero visits). While interpretation of the coefficients is more abstract, the results produced smaller standard errors compared to other adjustment methods.[1] Nonetheless, the statistical significance of independent variables was the same, regardless of the adjustment technique used.

As was the case with the analytical model for making any access to medical care, residential instability factors were unrelated to the total number of annual medical visits (Table 6.4). Current stability was also unrelated to total visits. Other statistically significant factors in the models are discussed later in this chapter.

Overall, the findings support the notion that a history of residential instability is associated with how poor families are connecting to the health care system, but is unrelated to whether or not they access it, or how often.

Table 6.3: Multivariate Logistic Regression Models for No Medical Visits in the Last Year

	Mothers (N=543) OR[a] (95% CI[b])	Children (N=765) OR (95% CI)
Predisposing Factors		
Age	1.0 (1.0, 1.1)	1.1 (1.0, 1.2)**
Mother Prefers Speaking Spanish	0.9 (0.3, 2.3)	0.6 (0.3, 1.5)
Childhood Poverty	0.6 (0.2, 1.3)	0.9 (0.5, 1.8)
Mother Pregnant/New Mother in 1988	1.6 (0.7, 3.8)	1.2 (0.6, 2.4)
Family Size	1.1 (0.8, 1.4)	1.1 (0.9, 1.3)
Residential Instability		
Pre-Time 1 Mobility	0.8 (0.2, 2.7)	1.0 (0.6, 1.6)
Ever Used Shelter	1.0 (0.4, 2.3)	0.8 (0.4, 1.6)
Post-Time 1 Mobility	1.2 (0.6, 2.7)	0.6 (0.3, 1.1)
Family & Community Enabling Factors		
Residential Stability	0.6 (0.2, 1.3)	1.2 (0.6, 2.5)
Mother Currently Employed	2.4 (0.8, 7.2)	2.1 (0.8, 5.5)
Not on Public Assistance	0.6 (0.2, 1.8)	0.8 (0.3, 2.2)
Can't Afford Medical Care	2.0 (0.9, 4.6)	1.5 (0.8, 3.0)
No Regular Source of Care	4.6 (1.8,11.7)**	4.8 (1.8, 12.6)**
Hospital in Family's Neighborhood	0.9 (0.4, 2.1)	0.6 (0.3, 1.2)
Illness/Need Factors		
Nº chronic health problems	0.7 (0.6, 0.9)*	0.8 (0.5, 1.1)
Pregnant during last year	1.3 (0.5, 0.7)	-----

[a]OR: Odds Ratio of the likelihood of having no visits in the last year
[b]CI: confidence interval
*P < .05; ** P < .01

Table 6.4: Multivariate Regression Models for Annual Medical Visits

	Mothers[a] (N=506) Coefficient (95% CI[b])	Children[a] (N=708) Coefficient (95% CI)
Predisposing Factors		
Age	-0.0 (-0.0, 0.0)	-0.0 (-0.0, -0.0)*
Mother Prefers Speaking Spanish	0.2 (-0.0, 0.4)	0.1 (0.0, 0.3)*
Childhood Poverty	-0.1 (-0.3, 0.0)	-0.0 (-0.2, 0.1)
Mother Pregnant/New Mother in 1988	-0.2 (-0.4, 0.0)	0.1 (-0.0, 0.2)
Family Size	-0.1 (-0.1, -0.0)*	0.0 (-0.1, 0.0)
Residential Instability		
Pre-Time 1Mobility	0.2 (-0.1, 0.4)	0.0 (-0.1, 0.1)
Ever Used Shelter	0.0 (-0.2, 0.2)	-0.0 (-0.1, 0.2)
Post-Time 1 Mobility	-0.1 (-0.3, 0.1)	-0.1 (-0.2, 0.0)
Family & Community Enabling Factors		
Residential Stability	0.1 (-0.1, 0.3)	-0.0 (-0.1, 0.2)
Mother Currently Employed	-0.3 (-0.7, -0.0)*	-0.0 (-0.3, 0.2)
Not on Public Assistance	-0.1 (-0.3, 0.2)	-0.3 (-0.5, -0.0)*
Can't Afford Medical Care	0.0 (-0.2, 0.3)	-0.0 (-0.2, 0.1)
No Regular Source of Care	-0.5 (-0.9, -0.2)**	-0.3 (-0.7, 0.1)
Hospital in Family's Neighborhood	0.1 (-0.1, 0.3)	-0.0 (-0.1, 0.2)
Illness/Need Factors		
Nº. chronic health problems	0.2 (0.1, 0.2)**	0.3 (0.2, 0.4)**
Pregnant last year	0.4 (0.2, 0.6)**	-------
Constant	1.5 (1.0, 2.0)**	1.2 (0.8, 1.6)**

[a]The regression analyses were conducted using the natural log of the dependent visit variable.

[b]CI: confidence interval

*P < .05; ** P < .01

THE DURATION OF SHELTER & OTHER FACTORS OF THE SHELTER EXPERIENCE

Another aspect of the research was to examine whether the amount of time families spent in shelter was related to current health care use. Only those families who spent any time in shelter were part of a subset of multivariate analyses. In keeping with the exploratory nature of the study's examination of residential instability, a "threshold" approach was applied to define discrete categories for the duration of shelter. Recall that the average length of stay in shelter is about one year. From the large number of length of stay combinations tested on this originally continuous variable, only the extreme high and low cases of shelter stays produced significant differences in health care use from the bulk of family shelter stays. In other words, health care utilization patterns did not vary significantly whether a family stayed in shelter three, six or 18 months. Only families who stayed less than one month or more than two years in shelter had different source of care outcomes from the majority of families. The length of stay in shelter was unrelated to visit outcomes, for all periods tested in preliminary analyses.

These early analyses also demonstrated that few other aspects of the shelter experience are related to recent health care use. Specifically, two additional measures of the shelter experience were considered as control factors in the multivariate models. Along with the duration of shelter, they are defined below, with relative frequencies for each category. Each variable relates to the period that families spent in shelter, for all episodes of shelter use after the Time 1 interview. An episode is a stay in shelter that includes an absence of less than 30 days out of shelter; i.e., breaks of less than 30 days are part of one episode.

Factors of the Shelter Experience

The number of months families spent in shelter, including breaks of less than 30 days.

Less than 1 month (11%)
Between 1 and 24 months (78%)
More than 24 months (11%)

The number of shelters that families stayed in until their last episode ended.

3 or more (50%)
2 or less (50%)

The type of shelter families stayed in during their longest episode (see Appendix A for a description).

Tier I/congregate (15%)
Welfare hotel (57%)
Tier II/family center apartment (28%)

Neither the type of shelter, which reflects the qualitative experience of the shelter stay, nor the number of shelters in which families stayed, which is a proxy for mobility during homelessness, was related to health care use for the year prior to the Time 2 interviews. Thus they were not included in the multivariate analyses.

Regular Source of Care

Table 6.5 presents the *adjusted* (controlling for other predisposing, enabling and illness factors) relative risk ratios for short and long shelter stays resulting from mothers' and children's multivariate health care utilization models. While the length of time families spent in shelter was unrelated to mothers' source of care patterns, children of families who spent less than one month in shelter had more than five times the relative risk of using an ED or having no regular source of care. Because of the smaller sample size, however, caution must be exercised in interpreting this result, as evidenced by the wide confidence interval. An extremely long stay in shelter—more than two years—was associated with a slight decrease in the relative risk of children using a Community/Public Health clinic as a regular source of care.

Medical Care Visits

Just as having ever used shelter was unrelated to visit outcomes, so was an extremely long stay in shelter (results not shown). In fact, none of the mothers who used shelter for more than two years had gone without a medical visit in the last year. However, the multivariate results showed that mothers who spent less than one month in shelter had 7

Table 6.5: Adjusted Relative Risk Ratios of Shelter Duration from Multivariate Regular Source of Care Models

Duration of Shelter	Hospital OPD	Community/ PH Clinic	ED/No Reg. Source
	RRR[a] (95% CI[b])	RRR (95% CI)	RRR (95% CI)
Mothers (N=248)			
Base is between 1 & 24 months			
< 1 month	2.1 (0.6, 7.9)	3.1 (0.8, 12.2)	2.6 (0.6, 11.0)
> 24 months	1.6 (0.4, 6.1)	0.6 (0.1, 3.1)	1.6 (0.4, 6.8)
Children (N=377)			
Base is between 1 & 24 months			
< 1 month	3.6 (1.2, 11.4)	2.8 (0.9, 8.9)	5.3 (1.2, 22.5)*
> 24 months	1.0 (0.4, 2.8)	0.3 (0.1, 1.0)*	1.0 (0.3, 3.4)

[a]RRR: Relative Risk Ratio; comparison is to a Private Doctor/HMO

[b]CI: confidence interval

*P< .05; **P< .01; ***P< .001

times the odds (OR= 7.2, CI= 1.8, 29.4) of going without any medical visits in the last year, compared to the reference group of mothers who spent between one and 24 months in shelter. Again, it is important to keep in mind that because of the small size of this subgroup, the standard error is extremely large, as evidenced by the width of this confidence interval. The length of the shelter stay was wholly unrelated to whether children made any medical visits in the last year. Likewise, the length of stay in shelter was unrelated to the total number of medical visits for both mothers and children.

SUMMARY OF MULTIVARIATE FINDINGS ON SHELTER USE AND MOBILITY

The results of the multivariate analyses spell out two related themes. The first is that—in the language of the Behavioral Model of Health Services Use—ever-sheltered families appear *predisposed* to using safety net providers and not having a regular source of care, compared to never-sheltered families. Ever-sheltered families' current relationship with the health care system appears tied to their *history* of residential instability, but not to their direct experiences with the shelter system. While current residential stability somewhat mitigates dependence on emergency department use or not having a regular source of care, a history of residential instability has a stronger association with where poor families currently seek health care.

In addition, a high degree of pre-Time 1 mobility increased ever-sheltered families' relative risk of ED use or not having a regular source of care more than recent mobility did. The threshold for pre-Time 1 mobility was very high and applied to only 12 percent of families. For those who experienced it, however, the relationship to current sources of health care is highly significant. One question is why a high degree of post-Time 1 mobility (relative to the average for post-Time 1 mobility) appears to matter less than earlier mobility. Does such mobility, whether shelter- or residential-related, matter little compared to the disruption of simply being homeless?

The second theme is that the shelter experience itself does not appear to have negative health care consequences for ever-sheltered families. In fact, becoming homeless but not staying in shelter long enough to obtain an apartment was associated with relatively worse access, while spending an extremely long time in shelter was not. Contrary to the related hypotheses, the findings suggest that something about the families who did not "do their time" in shelter is associated with having access barriers to medical care, rather than a long stay in shelter having a residual influence on families' capacity to access health care services appropriately, after leaving shelter. The results dispute notions that either a typical or extremely long shelter experience leads to long-term consequences for homeless families, regarding their use of health care services.

While not contradicting previous research findings on homeless families living in shelter, the results of this study suggest that health care utilization differences between ever-sheltered and never-sheltered families may have preceded entry into shelter. Unfortunately, we have no direct means to test this hypothesis. However, if this hypothesis were true, it would provide one plausible explanation for why ever-sheltered families, even after the vast majority are no longer homeless, have usual source of care patterns that look very different from never-sheltered families, and quite similar to families living in shelter.

An alternative explanation is that disruptions in attachments to private doctors, during periods of shelter use and high mobility, make it difficult for mothers to return to their original providers. While in shelter, families might have been transported to hospital clinics or received specialized services provided in shelter. Perhaps a stigma of homelessness follows families after they leave shelter, making it difficult for them to connect with physicians and HMOs in their new neighborhood.

Finally, it must be noted how ever-sheltered and never-sheltered families appear alike in their use of health care. Residential factors were unrelated to whether or not families had any visits in the last year, or to their total annual volume of medical care. Overall, poor families, regardless of their shelter status, or even where they go for care, appear to use health care in amounts relative to their perceived need for medical care. With need factors as the strongest predictors of the volume of care, these findings suggest that residential factors may not be a significant barrier to obtaining medical care. Medical need did not vary by shelter status, but perceived medical needs may not include preventive care. Because of their higher relative risk of not having a regular source of care or using an emergency department as a regular source of care, families who have left shelter may still not be obtaining adequate amounts of preventive care. Preventive care services are more difficult to come by through the emergency department or when one does not have a usual source of care that is an appropriate primary care provider.

In summary, a consistent pattern of insignificant associations between residential instability factors and the volume of medical care visits emerged from a number of models that utilized various analytical techniques and control variables. At the same time, when looking at several measures of residential instability across multiple models, the pattern of analytical findings points to the conclusion that a history of residential instability is highly related to where poor families currently seek health care.

Parenthetically, another series of multivariate analyses were conducted with a sample that excluded the eleven mothers still in shelter at Time 2. The results from those analyses produced almost identical results regarding the relationships between factors of residential instability and both regular sources of health care and visit outcomes.

OTHER FACTORS RELATED TO HEALTH CARE UTILIZATION

As expected, a number of control variables included in the analytical models were also statistically significant. These results are summarized below, as highlighted previously in Tables 6.1 and 6.2 for regular source of care outcomes, and Tables 6.3 and 6.4 for visit outcomes. Where significant findings were weak or inconsistent across mothers' and children's models, more caution must be exercised in making conclusions that may be a result of chance, particularly regarding small sub-groups of families with particular characteristics.

PREDISPOSING FACTORS

Age

Age was a significant factor in medical visit utilization among children, but not mothers. As children age from infancy to adolescence, they are more likely to go without medical care and average fewer total visits,[2] as the results here demonstrate. While this phenomenon tends to be true across the general population of children, it is of greater concern for children from both homeless and housed poor families because they have much higher rates of poor health and hospitalization than the general population.

Language

One of the strongest predisposing factors related to regular source of care for both mothers and children is a mother's preference for speaking Spanish (see Tables 6.1 and 6.2), described earlier as a proxy for acculturation with English-speaking communities. The results show that Spanish-speaking mothers and their children have a very low relative risk—10 percent—of using community/public health clinics over private doctors/HMOs. By contrast, 56 percent of all Spanish-speaking mothers, and 66 percent of their children, reported using a private doctor/HMO.

A lack of acculturation may be a result of language barriers, physical isolation, as well as the socio-political status of illegal residency, such that the relationship between preferring Spanish and source of care may be explained by a combination of individual perception and organizational orientation.[3] Spanish-speaking families are likely to seek care in places that are convenient to access, give them a sense of feeling welcome and not threatened, and allow them to speak their native language.[4] Medical settings that are culturally sensitive and/or provide translators are more likely to attract Spanish-speaking patients. Overall, private, office-based physicians may be less intimidating to Spanish-speaking families than institutional settings. The findings suggest that Spanish-speaking families may experience language or cultural barriers in accessing community health centers and health departments. Likewise, they may have relatively higher rates of private physician use because foreign-born medical school graduates, such as Dominican physicians, have established private practices that cater to neighborhoods with a high rate of Spanish-speaking Medicaid families.

Childhood Poverty & Pregnant or New Mother in 1988

Two of the strongest factors predicting a mother's request for shelter in 1988—childhood poverty and being pregnant or a new mother at Time 1—are also strongly associated with mothers having an increased relative risk of using community/public health clinics (RRR=2.1), and an ED/No regular source of care (RRR=3.1), respectively. These factors are not, however, associated with increased risks for children, suggesting that mothers may be more discerning about where they take their children for medical care than where they seek care for themselves. In fact, children of mothers with a history of welfare dependence have a significantly reduced risk of going to a hospital OPD over a private physician/HMO. Perhaps through their own experience with welfare as children or teens, they are familiar with private pediatricians who can care for their children.

At the same time, it remains a mystery as to why new motherhood in 1988 remains such a significant predictor of ED/No regular source of care for mothers years later. Could it be that many of these young women who became pregnant—and turned to the shelter system because they were no longer welcome at their family's residence and/or sought permanent housing via the shelter system queue—were disenfranchised from the mainstream health care system before becoming or while they were homeless? Perhaps they are continuing a reliance they established long ago.

Yet, being pregnant in the previous year is unrelated to current source of care utilization. Perhaps the experience of pregnancy in the context of more residential stability has less influence on a mother's perceived choices of where to obtain health care. On the other hand, pregnancy, itself, may simply not exert much influence on where poor mothers seek care, relative to where they obtained care before becoming pregnant. Wherever mothers go for care, however, recent pregnancy is significantly associated with an increase in the amount of care utilized in the last year, a positive indicator that suggests mothers are obtaining some measure of prenatal care, whether or not it is in an appropriate setting.

Family Size

As family size increases, so increases the relative risk of children having an emergency department as a regular source of care or not having one at all. This result is perhaps illustrating, in part, how the pressures of family circumstances may make an emergency department a convenient alternative for mothers to obtain non-emergency medical care for their children.

ENABLING FACTORS

Several enabling factors are associated with health care utilization for both mothers and children. Difficulty affording medical care is the one that most strongly relates to source of care patterns, and not having a regular source of care is highly predictive of total visits.

Currently Employed

Although only a small percentage—11 percent—of the entire sample was employed at Time 2, being employed reduced children's relative risk of using community/public health clinics over private doctors/HMOs as a regular source of care, suggesting that employment has an enabling effect on children's access to care. For mothers, however, employment was associated with a decrease in total visits, suggesting that the combined pressures of work and family may make it difficult to obtain time off to seek medical care.

Public Assistance and Problems Affording Medical Care

Mothers no longer on public assistance have 2.5 times the relative risk of using an ED/No regular source of care over private physicians/HMOs. A lack of public assistance is also associated with a decrease in the total number of medical visits among children, even after adjusting for illness levels and other factors. This finding is consistent with the health care utilization literature regarding the important enabling effects of Medicaid.[5]

At the same time, public assistance, through Medicaid, may be a necessary but insufficient means for poor families to gain appropriate access to health care. Even after controlling for public assistance status, the children of mothers who said that they often or very often could not afford medical care, have more than five times the relative risk—the strongest of any other children's factor—of using an ED or not having a regular source of care. Mothers themselves had more than three times this relative risk. These findings match with studies demonstrating a strong association between income and utilization, even after controlling for public assistance.[6] Thus, even with public assistance and Medicaid, a lack of financial means (or at least the perception of it) may lead poor families to greater reliance on emergency departments or to lack a regular source of care altogether.

Among mothers who reported no longer being on public assistance, 58 percent reported not having Medicaid and 42 percent reported they did have Medicaid, which is not directly measured in the public assistance variable. Surprisingly, mothers explicitly without Medicaid did not have a significantly higher relative risk of using an ED/No regular source of care, compared to those with Medicaid. The loss of income assistance and rental subsidies resulting from a closed welfare case may influence a mother's perception of affordability for medical care even more than the loss of Medicaid itself, considering the strong role that perceptions of affordability play, even when a family does have Medicaid coverage by virtue of being on public assistance.

No Regular Source of Care

Fortunately, only a minority of mothers and an even smaller percentage of children went without medical visits in the last year. Few variables were predictive of this rare event, but the strongest, by far, was whether one had a regular source of care. After illness levels and medical need, not having a regular source of care was the strongest predictor of mothers' total number of annual visits.

Community Resources

Having a hospital in a neighborhood doubles the relative risk of children using a hospital outpatient department or an ED/No regular source of care. While a nearby hospital seems to represent increased convenience for families to obtain health care for their children, more physicians—as evidenced in preliminary analyses—did not detract them away from hospital-based care. Thus, the presence of a neighborhood hospital appears to be an enabling factor, whether as an emergency or outpatient department, in providing a relatively accessible place for mothers to take their children for medical care.

Medical Needs

As expected, based on the health care utilization literature described earlier, the level of illness, defined here as the number of chronic health problems reported, is highly associated with health care use. For example, for each increase in the number of chronic conditions, the relative risk of mothers using hospital OPDs over private physicians/HMOs increases by 13 percent (RRR=1.13). Hospital-based clinics are more likely to provide specialty care than are the private physicians to whom poor families tend to have access.

As the number of chronic health conditions increases, the relative risk of using an ED or having no regular source of care drops significantly (RRR=0.83, mothers; RRR=0.62, children), suggesting that family members with serious health problems are obtaining some level of continuity of care for their illnesses. In the same vein, the more health problems family members have, the less likely they are to go without medical care altogether. Likewise, for each unit increase in the number of chronic health conditions, the total number of expected annual visits rises significantly.

As discussed earlier, being pregnant during the year prior to the Time 2 interview is also highly associated with the total number of mothers' visits. However, given the worse birth outcomes for ever-sheltered mothers, and the finding that pregnancy is not associated with a reduced risk of ED use/No regular source of care, it may be that some ever-sheltered mothers are not obtaining prenatal care in an appropriate setting.

The positive association between medical need and use, a widely reported finding in studies of the poor and non-poor alike, has been used to argue that our health care system is equitable.[7] Indeed, only 7 percent of mothers reported there was ever a time in the last year that they did not get care they needed; less than 3 percent reported that there was such a time for their children. Yet, one-fifth of all mothers reported having trouble affording medical care. Thus, poor mothers appear to be making health care seeking decisions based on medical need—and more. Poor urban families in New York City seem to be adapting their health care utilization behavior—and expectations—to the enabling circumstances of their own family and neighborhood resources, and to their prior experience with the health care system.

Ways in which policy makers might make adjustments as well, based on the implications of these research findings, are discussed in the next chapter.

NOTES

1. Li, G. (1985). Robust Regression. In D. C. Hoaglin, F. Mosteller, & J. Tukey (Eds.), *Exploring Data Tables, Trends, Trends and Shapes* (pp. 281-340). New York: John Wiley & Sons.

2. Kleinman, J. C., Gold, M., & Makuc, D. (1981). Use of ambulatory medical care by the poor: Another look at equity. *Medical Care*, 19 (10), 1011-1029.

3. Lewin-Epstein, N. (1991). Determinants of regular source of health care in Black, Mexican, Puerto Rican, and Non-Hispanic white populations. *Medical Care*, 29 (6), 543-557.

4. Ibid.

5. Marquis, M. S. & Long, S. H. (1996). Reconsidering the effect of Medicaid on health services use. *Health Services Research*, 30 (6), 791-807.

6. Dutton, D. B. (1978). Explaining the low use of health services by the poor: Costs, attitudes, or delivery systems? *American Sociological Review*, 43 (6), 348-368.

7. Wolinsky, F. D. (1978). Assessing the effects of predisposing, enabling and illness-morbidity characteristics on health service utilization. *Journal of Health and Social Behavior*, 19, 384-396.

CHAPTER 7

Program and Policy Recommendations to Improve Health Care Access

MANY FAMILIES LACK AN APPROPRIATE MEDICAL HOME AFTER HOMELESSNESS

The residential stability that most formerly homeless families will achieve offers a chance to develop a long-term relationship with an appropriate health care provider. The results of this study suggest that many of these families, however, are missing this opportunity. Formerly homeless families are likely to maintain relatively weak links to mainstream health care providers, without some form of programmatic effort to change this pattern. This may be all the more likely if current health care use is a continuation of patterns preceding shelter use. Even without the data to show such a continuation, the implications are the same: policy makers are missing an opportunity to improve health care access for a population that has a relatively high risk of not having a regular source of care or an appropriate one, and yet can easily be identified and targeted for intervention.

Further supporting the notion of missed opportunities are the relatively worse birth outcomes among ever-sheltered families. Birth outcomes are considered sensitive indicators of access to primary care, and are strongly correlated with prenatal care visits.[1] For all three of the birth statistics mothers were asked to report on, children born to ever-sheltered mothers had worse outcomes than children born to never-sheltered mothers. The consistency of outcomes across age groups may indicate that access to prenatal care will not improve for mothers after homelessness, without interventions to improve their overall access to appropriate health care providers.

SAFETY NET PROVIDERS ARE CRUCIAL PLAYERS IN HEALTH CARE DELIVERY TO POOR FAMILIES

Safety net providers play a vital role in filling the gaps left by the private sector. Fully, 60 percent of mothers rely on providers other than private physicians/HMOs, with about one-third of both ever- and never-sheltered families using hospital outpatient departments (OPDs) as a regular source of care. As the number of chronic health problems a mother has increases, so does the relative risk that she will use a hospital OPD over a private physician/HMO as a regular source of care. In addition, neighborhood hospitals seem to provide families a convenient source of access to health care, either through outpatient clinics or emergency departments. Poor families are likely to remain solid users of hospital-based sources of care, without a lack of convenient alternatives. Regarding HMOs, this means having a well-developed, culturally sensitive physician network.

LONG-TERM SHELTER USERS DO NOT FARE WORSE THAN OTHER SHELTERED FAMILIES

Neither a long shelter stay, nor other aspects of shelter use were related to families' current health care utilization patterns. On the contrary, only the minority of families who stayed less than a month in shelter appeared to underutilize health care, relative to other sheltered families. The family shelter system, itself, does not appear to be creating or extending barriers to health care beyond the shelter experience. In fact, the results raise questions about whether the patterns exhibited by families while they are living in shelter, as documented in studies described earlier, were already established, to some extent, before entering shelter. The implication is that the shelter experience will neither worsen nor reduce the barriers families face in establishing appropriate health care relationships after leaving shelter. The results also raise questions about whether specialized services to homeless families may even disrupt ties to mainstream providers. Policies designed to lessen health care access barriers for homeless families are inadequate for addressing the barriers families face after leaving the shelter system.

POVERTY, BUT NOT HOMELESSNESS IS RELATED TO POOR FAMILIES' HEALTH STATUS

Despite differences found in birth outcomes, children of ever-sheltered families have rates of chronic health problems and levels of fair/poor health status, as well as health care visit and hospitalization rates, almost identical to those of never-sheltered children. When adjusted for age, ever-sheltered and never-sheltered mothers do not differ significantly on rates of fair/poor health status or chronic illnesses, nor on the amount of health care they use. Even death rates are similar, with AIDS being the leading cause of death for both samples of mothers. As a whole, poor families have dramatically higher chronic illness and health care utilization rates than the general population. Such findings further underscore the role of poverty—including deficient housing, environmental, and dietary conditions—on the health status of poor, American families. Homelessness may be an extreme form of poverty, but for most it is a temporary decline in an otherwise continuing cycle of inadequate resources and too few opportunities.

Policies limited to maintaining adequate living standards for families while they are living in shelter help in the short-term, at best. They have little long-term value in promoting a healthy and safe living environment for families after they leave the shelter system, or in preventing the conditions that lead to homelessness for some and poor health for so many. As long as the conditions of poverty exist—even if homelessness were eradicated—poor families will continue to have a higher need for health care services than the general population. There is tremendous need for *all* poor families, not just those who are the temporary responsibility of a shelter system, to have safe housing, a healthy environment and appropriate access to high quality health care services.

PUBLIC ASSISTANCE IS NOT ENOUGH, BUT IT HELPS

Even among those with Medicaid coverage, the affordability of health care is a significant factor in mothers' health care decision-making. At the same time, not being on public assistance increases the relative risk of ED use/No regular source of care for mothers, and reduces the expected number of health care visits among children. Efforts to increase the cost burden to Medicaid-covered families, such as charging or increasing co-payments, or policies that limit poor families' access to public assistance or Medicaid are likely to increase the risk of poor families using an emergency department and not being able to maintain a regular source of health care.

POLICY RECOMMENDATIONS

Any set of recommendations responding to these research findings and implications must address the rapidly changing landscape of health care and welfare policies affecting poor families. For example, across the country, managed care has emerged as the major strategy for delivering health care to families on welfare.[2] By mid-1997, more than 15 million—almost one-half—of 32 million Medicaid recipients were in a managed care arrangement, according to the Health Care Financing Administration.[3] Since 1992, Medicaid managed care enrollment has increased by more than 170 percent, making HCFA the nation's largest purchaser of managed care.[4] In 1995, almost two of every three privately insured Americans were enrolled in a managed care plan.[5] Today, 85 percent of all workers are enrolled in some form of managed care.[6]

Currently, 17 states, including New York, have obtained Medicaid "1115 waivers" from HCFA to become exempt from Social Security laws that would otherwise prevent states from mandating Medicaid beneficiaries to enroll in a managed care plan or limit beneficiaries' choice of provider.[7] The primary goal of states, by implementing their Medicaid waivers, is to reduce the growth of their Medicaid budgets, while having the discretion to expand Medicaid coverage to previously uninsured populations, namely the working poor, who make up the vast majority of the uninsured.[8,9]

In 1991, New York State passed legislation requiring local social services agencies to develop a managed care program for Medicaid recipients.[10] In the absence of the waiver, which, at the time of this writing, has yet to be implemented, the state turned to voluntary enrollment of welfare recipients into managed care health plans. New York and other states or localities that have implemented Medicaid managed care—whether voluntarily, or with a mandate—have faced a barrage of concern and criticism about managed care's effects on health care access and quality for vulnerable populations.[11–15]

Some of those concerns are beginning to be realized, as several commercial health plans have begun pulling out of Medicaid managed care markets in New York and other northeastern states, citing state reductions in reimbursement as the primary cause of the decision to withdraw from the program.[16] A recent study by the Inspector General of the Department of Health and Human Services found that less than one-third of children enrolled in managed care were receiving timely preventive care screenings and 60 percent received none at all.[17] At the same time, safety net providers in the most underserved urban communities, which have traditionally used Medicaid reimbursement to subsidize care to the uninsured, are losing substantial revenues from Medicaid clients who sign up for managed care health plans.[18] More community clinics are closing or barely surviving, leaving uninsured clients with greatly reduced access to primary care.

Predicting the ultimate consequences of Medicaid managed care is complicated by legislation recently passed by Congress to set time limits on welfare entitlements. The "Personal Responsibility and Work Opportunity Reconciliation Act of 1996" ended the federal guarantee of cash assistance to poor children, replacing Aid to Families with Dependent Children (AFDC), with Temporary Assistance to Needy Families (TANF).[19] Two major provisions of the federal bill are to require heads of TANF households to work within two years, or lose benefits, and to limit lifetime welfare benefits to five years (with hardship exemptions available for 20 percent of families).

Welfare rolls have begun shrinking dramatically around the country as the law takes effect.[20] In New York alone, the drop in the last three years is more than 30 percent, to 797,000.[21] Recent studies indicate that only about half of mothers leaving welfare find part-time or full-time employment, typically at low wages—which keeps them well in poverty's reach.[22] The other half pieces together support from family, friends and short-term work stints. While the children of former welfare families who still earn low incomes are entitled to remain on Medicaid, mothers have to make a special effort to apply. Federal estimates are that 3 million children—one-third of all uninsured children—were eligible for but not enrolled in Medicaid in 1997, and the gap is projected to rise as welfare rolls continue to drop.[23] The situation has led federal officials to call for increased efforts, nationwide, to identify and enroll eligible children into Medicaid. However, identifying those eligible children, whose parents are no longer part of the welfare system that once tracked them, poses substantial challenges.

Welfare reform also includes limits on benefits, including Medicaid, to legal immigrants, which may further expand the size of the uninsured population. The increased demands made on safety net providers, particularly in New York, California, Florida and Texas, where immigrant populations are most concentrated, may lead to more unmet health needs for both uninsured and Medicaid families who depend on community clinics and public hospitals.[24] Many of these providers, especially in the most underserved communities, are facing closure or severe down-sizing as they struggle with the shift of Medicaid dollars to managed care plans.

The intersection of Medicaid managed care and welfare reform is presenting momentous challenges to policy makers, community-based health providers and poor families nationwide. Fortunately, new funds have recently become available for states to extend Medicaid coverage or create a new state children's health insurance program (S-CHIP) for children from households with too much income to qualify previously for Medicaid benefits.[25] The program was created in the Balanced Budget Act of 1997, in part, as a response to census data showing that about 14 percent of the nation's children under 18 years of age were uninsured in 1995.[26]

The S-CHIP program is expected to increase insurance coverage up to five million children, half of the estimated uninsured children in the U.S., yet it does not expand coverage for uninsured parents or adults,[27] thus maintaining a fragmented system of health care access for poor families. The new program funding has the potential to provide better access to mainstream health care for a vulnerable portion of the uninsured population, but it still makes only a dent in reducing the swelling ranks of the uninsured, currently estimated at 41.4 million, according to the Employee Benefit Research Institute.[28] President Clinton's recent proposal to allow uninsured individuals between 55 and 65 to buy into Medicare is noble, but still ignores a significant portion of the uninsured. Thus, it seems that working-poor parents with school-age children are the lowest on the totem pole for government assistance with health insurance.

Based on the current health policy environment and the implications of the research results presented, I propose the following recommendations, summarized below:

1. Increase the opportunities for families leaving shelter to enroll in Medicaid managed care.
2. Require managed care plans to be more accountable for managing the health needs and conditions of poor families, particularly those with chronic illnesses.
3. Require managed care plan plans to be more accountable for improving the health and health-related conditions of poor communities.
4. Maintain adequate financial support of safety net providers, even as Medicaid managed care enrollment expands.
5. Provide universal access to health insurance coverage to improve the chances of achieving the goals of both managed care and welfare reform.

HELP FAMILIES FIND A MEDICAL HOME AFTER HOMELESSNESS

New York and other urban cities need a proactive approach to ensure that formerly homeless families do not remain marginalized from mainstream health care providers, particularly at a time when the health care system is undergoing vast, structural changes. The changes include more privatization of health care services to the poor, and more community-based providers starting their own managed care plans or contracting with private plans. By connecting soon-to-be formerly homeless families with managed care plans, whether privately or publicly managed, cities could help expand managed care enrollment to a segment of the Medicaid population that is relatively more reliant on emergency departments and less likely to have a regular source care. In purely social terms, families could very well benefit from the attention they would receive as a card-carrying health care consumer, just as they are starting Life After Shelter.

Efforts by appropriate government and/or private agencies could be coordinated such that families leaving shelter for a new apartment have an opportunity to learn about managed care concepts and meet with plan representatives about potential providers in the neighborhood to which they will be moving. Without this coordination being provided while the "system" is still keeping track of them, many formerly homeless families are likely to continue using an emergency department as their entry point for primary care services, or to continue relying on an "unmanaged" mix of hospital outpatient departments and community clinics, where they may have difficulty establishing an on-going physician-patient relationship.

As proposed, health plans would have a formal process for recruiting a segment of the Medicaid population that is typically younger and as healthy or healthier than the welfare population as a whole. This coordination serves an educational purpose for health plan administrators, who may have misconceptions about the characteristics and needs of (formerly) homeless families. Once health plans know some of the comparative information about homeless and housed welfare families, they might eagerly participate in arrangements for targeted enrollment of families exiting shelter.

Nonetheless, it must be acknowledged that sheltered families may over-represent welfare families who are vulnerable to managed care access problems.[29] For example, formerly homeless families may have relatively more difficulty following the strict rules on emergency department use because they are relatively more dependent on them for primary care. They may also have more difficulty making the transition to mandatory enrollment in Medicaid managed care. Targeted managed care education and support for formerly homeless families could greatly increase the likelihood that managed care lives up to its promise of helping poor families establish an on-going physician-patient relationship. Managed care policies related to homeless families should focus on empowerment, not protectionism, while simultaneously making health plans more accountable to poor families as a whole.

In New York City, managed care organizations (MCOs) have been required to exclude homeless families from enrollment in their programs.[30] Living in shelter is itself grounds for disenrollment from Medicaid managed care. The City's objective is to avoid paying the capitated premium to a health plan and simultaneously paying the Medicaid fees for care provided at emergency rooms or by shelter-based providers that are outside of the health plan's network.[31] Within its request for a federal Medicaid waiver, New York State proposed that families who enter shelter enroll in a city-wide Medicaid managed care plan, or switch to one, if they are already enrolled in a borough-wide plan.[32] In New York City, at least, enrollment in Medicaid managed care will remain voluntary for sheltered welfare clients, even after the federal Medicaid waiver is implemented.[33]

These policies are fine as far as they go; they simply do not go far enough. Even providers for Health Care for the Homeless, who treat primarily homeless individuals, speak of a philosophy to "provide acute care to their clients and then to attempt to mainstream them into established health care systems."[34] Homeless families as well, when they leave shelter, need to be mainstreamed into established health care systems, which increasingly will mean a managed care arrangement.

IMPROVE THE ACCOUNTABILITY OF MANAGED CARE ORGANIZATIONS TO POOR FAMILIES

Both the fee-for-service system of traditional Medicaid and the capitated payment system of managed care produce tendencies to hinder access.[35,36] Unlike traditional Medicaid, pre-paid health plans require patient registration with a physician or physician group. This offers the potential for greater accountability to both patients and payers, in part, through mandatory benefits, state and industry performance standards, and access to a primary care provider.[37] In practice, standards of care are often lacking or are not enforced, and provider shortages remain a serious problem in the inner cities.[38–41]

The need for better accountability from health plans is a special concern for the chronically ill poor, a category befitting many families on public assistance. Ware, et al. found that poor patients in HMOs, particularly the chronically ill among them, were at significantly greater risk for a decline in health compared to similar patients in a fee-for-service plan.[42] The high level of fair/poor health status found among the families of this study highlights the need to evaluate the quality of Medicaid managed care plans by patient health status or case mix. Most of the systems currently used for evaluating care, however, have focused not on distributions, but on averages, which exaggerate negative incentives to enroll high-risk or sick patients.[43] More research is needed to develop quality measures and payment systems that are adequately risk-adjusted, so that health plans have stronger incentives to provide quality health care to poor and chronically ill populations.[44]

In fact, to achieve long-term reductions in health care spending increases—part of the promise of managed care—policies and managed care practices must produce market forces that reconfigure the existing medical infrastructure. The transformation must be to a primary care model that provides long-term, continuous treatment to those with long-term, continuous illnesses, rather than treating chronic illnesses as a series of "separate, acute episodes."[45] With the disabled and long-term care populations consuming 59 percent of all Medicaid spending,[46] there is growing pressure for states to enroll these populations into managed care. Disabled and chronically ill populations present enormous challenges and opportunities to managed care organizations to shape a primary care model of health care delivery that improves the quality of health care for those who need health care the most. *Mandatory* enrollment of the chronically ill and disabled into managed care is a growing trend as well, although it is still not the dominant approach. By early 1996, 17 states had implemented prepaid managed care programs for disabled Medicaid beneficiaries, with six operating as a mandatory program.[47]

The art and science of risk-adjustment have advanced significantly with the recent development of health-based payment systems, which are intended to set payment rates that allow health plans to compete on value instead of risk-selection.[48] Some states are experimenting with an innovative strategy, called "risk-corridors," to reduce both cherry-picking the healthiest patients and underserving the sickest.[49] The strategy limits profits as well as losses to a health plan, by sharing both, between the state and the payer, within certain percentage rates or corridors. Others are employing a Disability Payment System that utilizes 400 distinct diagnoses to create a rate adjustment factor for individual patients that can account for multiple diagnoses. States should continue to develop and test these risk-adjustment systems with appropriate research evaluation, such that their effectiveness can be measured and the lessons learned can be shared with other states.

IMPROVE THE ACCOUNTABILITY OF MANAGED CARE ORGANIZATIONS TO POOR COMMUNITIES

Managed care as *mainstream* health care should not be confused with *ideal* health care for poor families. Language and cultural barriers, not having a telephone, violent neighborhoods, poor nutrition, high rates of chronic conditions, such as asthma, diabetes and hypertension, along with poor access to affordable, high quality produce—all in addition to living in a medically underserved community—are concerns that transcend homelessness. But they also make providing managed care for welfare or other low-income families different from doing so for middle class families.[50–52] The improvements that the health care system can make to poor families' health, of course, are limited by the many non-medical factors of poverty.

While it is unrealistic to expect MCOs to eradicate poverty from urban neighborhoods, it is appropriate to expect them to return a dividend to the communities in which they have prospered. Much of their prosperity, in fact, has been forged on "an existing medical infrastructure funded by taxpayer dollars for the development of biomedical knowledge and technologies, training of health professionals, and construction of health care facilities."[53] A dividend should come by way of accountability for community-based outcomes rather than health outcomes only for the plan's enrolled members. Accountability requires MCOs to compete on outcomes, services and convenience, and to collaborate with community-based providers and other health plans to develop a network for collecting and sharing information on their financial performance and contributions to community health improvements.

Community-based providers are typically experienced in providing "enabling" services to address transportation, language and cultural barriers, with their long history of serving Medicaid and other poor populations, often in communities with few providers.[54] For managed care to reign as a cost-effective alternative to traditional fee-for-service care in poor, underserved communities, it may be imperative that managed care organizations collaborate with community-based organizations.

However, as the managed care industry grows and matures, and still struggles with its role in poor communities, some of the largest and most profitable commercial plans have recently chosen to drop their Medicaid business altogether. This growing phenomenon is raising strong concerns about many health plans' accountability to the states and communities that funded them, and the members who chose a primary care doctor from their network.[55] A cut in monthly per member premiums in the tri-state area of New York, New Jersey, and Connecticut has been blamed for the withdrawals from Medicaid. New York State's 1997 weighted average monthly premiums dropped by 22 percent from 1994 to 1997, according to the New York State Health Maintenance Organization Conference and Council. Advocates for the poor predict that when private providers are ill-equipped or otherwise not held accountable to care for the chronically ill poor, those patients will fall back on the health care safety net.[56] Findings from this study suggest that they already do; many poor mothers with chronic illnesses turn to hospital outpatient departments as their regular source of care.

In some cases, public hospitals, themselves, are developing their own Medicaid managed care plans,[57] just as a number of commercial plans are beginning to shrink from Medicaid programs. Increasingly, non-profit community providers and traditional safety net institutions that already serve vulnerable populations, such as the homeless, mentally ill and severely disabled, have restructured in some capacity to participate directly in managed care.[58,59] These organizations have accepted risk-arrangements that will funnel existing public funds to their programs, in exchange for managing the physical, mental and/or psycho-social health of those they currently serve. While the managed care revolution has already forced many safety net providers to become more fiscally efficient, these fledgling community-based MCOs lack the experience of traditional MCOs in claims processing, provider relations, utilization review and financial risk management.[60]

Both could benefit from collaboration. Needless to say, the contracting issues are complex because they must address a broad set of issues, ranging from the scope of services to payment arrangements, to quality assurance and reporting requirements. These new structures and alliances will need adequate financing, community support and strong leadership to flourish. As they become more sophisticated in their financing, information and patient care management, we may see a "mainstreaming" of vulnerable populations into managed care partnerships that can provide higher quality health care more effectively than either a traditional safety net provider or a traditional health plan can alone.[61]

Policy makers can play a vital role in promoting such collaborations, which may be necessary to ensure the continued participation of commercial MCOs in Medicaid managed care, and to assure the survival of safety net providers. Policies should focus on maintaining adequate levels of payment to plans, in part, through more sophisticated risk-adjusted rates. This is also likely to increase the incentive for MCOs to collaborate with community-based providers, who they may perceive as treating only high-risk populations.[62]

Failed attempts in Newark, New Jersey offer a cautionary tale for policy makers, and safety net providers who attempt to compete or collaborate with managed care plans. The goal was to develop a managed care plan among community-based providers in the state. Instead, four community health clinics that served Medicaid clients and the uninsured have closed since New Jersey implemented mandatory Medicaid managed care.[63] Because many community-based providers may not have the managed care experience and financial reserves necessary to meet state requirements for HMO licensing, legislation is needed to generate incentives among both MCOs and community-based providers to collaborate. For example, legislation could allow providers to share automatically in the savings they may generate for MCOs from collaborating with them.[64]

MAINTAIN ADEQUATE SUPPORT FOR SAFETY NET PROVIDERS

As commercial health plans pull out of the Medicaid market and community providers struggle to fill the gaps and expand to populations that traditional MCOs have avoided, the necessity of safety net providers to the success and accountability of Medicaid managed care becomes increasingly clear. Just as crucial is the role that community-based providers play as providers of last resort for the uninsured and other vulnerable populations. Access to health care for the uninsured has become more difficult as competition for paying patients intensifies among both public and private providers.[65] Safety net providers that compete for scarce Medicaid managed care dollars may find it increasingly difficult to continue cost-shifting Medicaid dollars to the uninsured, as they traditionally have done under fee-for-service arrangements.

In many states, Medicaid managed care is resulting in a shift of disproportionate share hospital (DSH) funding away from subsidizing uncompensated hospital care, towards expanding Medicaid coverage to a greater portion of the uninsured poor.[66] But improved access for some comes at the expense of those who remain uninsured, in part, because this shift would occur even if Medicaid managed care does not lead to lower costs to safety net institutions.[67] Gold, Sparer and Chu note that stress on the safety net from DSH transfers is more likely to "have a negative effect in cities such as New York and Los Angeles, where large public systems play a major role."[68] Unlike California, with its explicit strategy to protect safety net institutions, New York delegated each county to develop its own managed care initiative, leaving safety net providers to fend for themselves.[69]

In New York City, voluntary Medicaid managed care is being implemented as the public hospital system is being down-sized through extensive layoffs and other cost-cutting measures.[70] However, New York City's Health and Hospital Corporation recently announced that it is expected to receive $500 million of $1.25 billion in additional Medicaid funding, as part of the waiver agreement mandating Medicaid managed care enrollment in New York State.[71] The funds are intended to help the local health care union's workers and non-profit hospitals with a high rate of Medicaid patients make the transition to managed care, through the expansion of outpatient services and worker retraining.

Paradoxically, as Medicaid managed care grows, so too grows communities' dependence on safety net institutions as providers of last resort. For these reasons, policy makers must protect the viability of safety net providers even as they implement Medicaid managed care. Shifting large amounts of DSH funds away from institutions to expand Medicaid coverage, without reinvesting some of it to preserve the viability of safety net providers, may do more harm than good. This may be especially true if health plans have not yet built enough provider capacity in poor neighborhoods or collaborated fairly with community providers, or their accountability to the state is weak.

EXPAND MEDICAID COVERAGE TOWARDS ENACTING UNIVERSAL HEALTH INSURANCE

Poor families' dependence on safety net providers may become even more pronounced as new welfare reforms to move TANF adults from welfare to work are implemented. Researchers have predicted a sizable increase in the number of uninsured in Wisconsin, as a result of welfare reforms already underway.[72,73] Ironically, the least likely or prepared to obtain gainful employment within a two year limit are long-term welfare recipients.[74] They are over-represented by minority women, with low levels of education and little, recent work experience, who become dependent on welfare at a young age.[75]

The sampling strategy of this research introduced a bias towards long-term welfare recipients by requiring that respondents—whether housed or requesting shelter—be receiving public assistance (or have a pending case) in order to be interviewed in 1988. The Urban Institute projects that "women who *ever* use welfare will receive assistance for about six years and *current* recipients will receive assistance for about thirteen years."[76] Of the mothers comprising the present study, 78 percent were still on public assistance four to five years after their initial interview.

Health problems may be a significant factor in the lack of employment among long-term welfare recipients. While overall employment for the Time 2 sample was low, unemployed mothers were almost twice as likely to be in fair or poor health compared to employed mothers (43% v. 23%). Likewise, more than twice as many unemployed mothers than employed mothers had at least one child in fair or poor health (19% v. 9%). Moffit and Wolfe found that Medicaid's influence on labor and welfare participation was strongest among those with the highest expected medical expenditures.[77]

The results of a ten-state demonstration project designed to break the cycle of welfare dependency, unemployment, and repeated pregnancy among young, low income women, in fact, demonstrated the extreme difficulties impoverished families face in the rush to self-sufficiency.[78] After more than three years, the great majority of the experimental group remained both poor and on welfare, showing little difference on outcome measures. In fact, women in the experimental group were more depressed, suggesting that the program increased hopeful expectations of changes that never occurred. While both groups of women expressed initial interest in education, factors such as homelessness, violence in the home, inadequate transportation and child care eroded this interest over time. Concerns that employment might leave them without health insurance coverage grew over time as well.

Allowing former welfare-dependent and other poor, working mothers to stay on Medicaid, or maintain some form of health insurance—even if they earn incomes above the limits set for maintaining Medicaid eligibility (set at July, 1996 income levels according to HCFA)—is likely to improve the odds that welfare reform will succeed with the population that most challenges its policy objectives: long-term welfare mothers, many of whom suffer from chronic illness or disability. The new children's health insurance program, described earlier, and efforts to increase Medicaid enrollment among children already eligible are steps in the right direction, but they do not address the larger issue of a growing lack of health insurance coverage among working poor families—including parents. Continuous health insurance coverage—for all family members—is necessary, even if not sufficient, to break the cycle of poverty that daily challenges the lives of millions of poor families.

CONCLUSION

The confluence of state and local changes in Medicaid policy, with major changes in federal welfare policy, portends more uncertainty about health care access for poor families. Results from this study of poor New York City families, many of which are headed by long-term welfare recipients with chronic illnesses, highlight the promises and challenges of these bold, yet untested policies, to achieve their *intended* consequences: moving adults on welfare into employment and self-sufficiency; improving health care quality and access to poor families through managed care; and reducing the costs and size of the health care safety net. Perhaps an *unintended* consequence of these federal, state and local policy interactions will be that policy makers are compelled to enact legislation on universal health insurance, a crucial missing link to each of these policy goals. Many factors—affordable housing, safe neighborhoods, high-quality public education, and economic opportunities, to name a few—can play a significant role in reducing poverty and therefore improving health. In the meantime, universal health insurance coverage would go along way towards improving access to health care and the quality of life of our nation's poor families.

NOTES

1. Reed, W. L. (1990). Racism and health: The case of Black infant mortality, in P. Conrad and R. Kern (Eds.), *The Sociology of Health and Illness* (3rd ed., pp. 34-44). New York: St. Martin's Press.

2. Rowland, D., & Hanson, K. (1996). Medicaid: Moving to managed care. *Health Affairs*, 15 (3), 150-167.

3. Health Care Finance Administration [HCFA]. (1998, February 28). *National summary of Medicaid managed care programs and enrollment.* Baltimore, MD: US Department of Health and Human Services.

4. HCFA. (1997, August 19). Managed care in Medicare and Medicaid. *Fact Sheet.* Baltimore, MD: US Department of Health and Human Services.

5. Hellinger, F. J. (1996). The expanding scope of state legislation. *JAMA*, 276 (October 2), 1065-1070.

6. Kilborn, P. T. (1998, March 22). Looking back at Jackson Hole. *The New York Times*, p. 16.

7. Iglehart, J. K. (1995). Health policy report: Medicaid and managed care. *New England Journal of Medicine*, 332 (June 22), 1727-1731.

8. Holohan, J., Coughlin, T., Ku, L., Lipson, D. J., & Rajan, S. (1995). Insuring the poor through section 1115 Medicaid waivers. *Health Affairs*, 14 (1), 199-216.

9. Blumberg, L.J., & Liska, D. W. (1996). *The uninsured in the United States: A status report.* Washington, DC: The Urban Institute.

10. Sparer, M. S. (1996). Medicaid managed care and the health reform debate: Lessons from New York and California. *Journal of Health Politics, Policy, and Law*, 21 (3), 433-459.

11. Gold, M., Sparer, M., & Chu, K. (1996). Medicaid managed care: Lessons from five states. *Health Affairs*, 15 (3), 153-165.

12. Douglass, R. L., & Torres, R. E. (1994). Evaluation of a managed care program for the non-Medicaid urban poor. *Journal of Health Care for the Poor and Underserved*, 5, 83-97.

13. Wood, D., Halfron, N., Sherbourne, C., & Grabowsky, M. (1994). Access to infant immunizations for poor inner-city families: What is the impact of managed care? *Journal of Health Care for the Poor and Underserved*, 5 (2), 112-123.

14. Goldman, B. (1993). Improving access to the underserved through Medicaid managed care. *Journal of Health Care for the Poor and Underserved*, 4 (3), 290-308.

15. Gordon, S. (1996). *Removing barriers, improving choices: A case study on reproductive health services in managed care settings.* New York: Center for Reproductive Law & Policy.

16. Fisher, I. (1998, February 26). HMO drops Medicaid in Connecticut. *The New York Times*, pp. 1, 6.

17. Pear, R. (1997, December 29). Clinton ordering effort to sign up Medicaid children. *The New York Times*, pp. 1, 15.

18. Goldstein, A. (1998, January 3). Clinics losing ground in drive toward managed care. *The Washington Post*, pp. 1, 10, 11.

19. HCFA. (1996). *National summary of Medicaid managed care programs and enrollment as of June 30 of each year*. Baltimore, MD: US Department of Health and Human Services.

20. DeParle, J. (1996, October 20). Slamming the door. *The New York Times Magazine*, pp. 52-63.

21. Toy, V. S. (1998, April 15). Tough workfare rules used as way to cut welfare rolls. *The New York Times*, pp. 1, B4.

22. Urban Institute. (1997, November). *Welfare recipients and work: What can be expected?* (Issue No. 27, Update). Washington, DC: Author.

23. Pear, R. (1997, December 29).

24. Baxter, R. J., & Mechanic, R. E. (1997). The status of local health care safety nets. *Health Affairs*, 16 (4), 7-23.

25. Urban Institute. (1998). *Health insurance for US children: Ten basic questions answered*. Washington, DC: Author.

26. Weil, A. (1997, October). *The new children's health insurance program: Should states expand Medicaid?* (No. A-13 in series, New federalism: Issues and options for states). Washington, DC: Urban Institute.

27. Urban Institute. (1998).

28. Kilborn, P. T. (1998, March 22).

29. Mayor's Advisory Council on Child Health. (1993). *Medicaid managed care in New York City: How will children fare?* New York: Child Health Action Management Plan.

30. Ibid.

31. S. Wiviott, Director of Policy, New York City Department of Homeless Services, personal communication, July 15, 1996.

32. State of New York. (1995). *The Partnership Plan*. Presented to the Secretary of Health and Human Services and the Administration of the Health Care Financing Administration, Albany, NY: Author.

33. Office of Medicaid Managed Care. (1996, June). *Medicaid model contract for fully capitated managed care providers under the Partnership Plan*. New York: Medicaid Assistance Program, City of New York.

34. Cousineau, M. R., Wittenberg, E., & Pollatsek, J. (1995). *A study of the health care for the homeless program*. Report to U.S. Department of Health and Human Services, Public Health Service, Health Resources and Services Administration, Bureau of Primary Health Care, Special Populations Division, p. 88.

35. Frederick Schneiders Research. (1996). *Medicaid and managed care: Focus group studies of low-income Medicaid beneficiaries in five states* (Report prepared for the Henry J. Kaiser Family Foundation). Washington, DC: Author.

36. Davis, K., & Rowland, D. (1991). Financing health care for the poor. In E. Ginzberg (Ed.), *Health Services Research*. Cambridge, MA: Harvard University Press, 93-125.

37. Bodenheimer, T. S., & Grumbach, K. (1996). Capitation or decapitation. *JAMA*, 276 (October 2), 1025-1031.

38. General Accounting Office [GAO]. (1997). *Medicaid Managed Care: The challenge of holding plans accountable requires greater state effort* (Report No. GAO/HEHS-97-86). Washington, DC: US Government Printing Office.

39. Gordon, S. (1996). *Removing barriers, improving choices: A case study on reproductive health services in managed care settings*. New York: Center for Reproductive Law & Policy.

40. Iglehart, J. K. (1995). Health policy report: Medicaid and managed care. *New England Journal of Medicine*, 332 (June 22), 1727-1731.

41. Light, D. W. (1994). Managed care: False and real solutions. *The Lancet*, 344 (October 29), 1197-1199.

42. Ware, J. E., Bayliss, M. S., Rogers, W. H., Kosinski, M., & Tarlov, A. R. (1996). Differences in 4-year health outcomes for elderly and poor, chronically ill patients treated in HMO and fee-for-service systems. *JAMA*, 276 (October 2), 1039-1047.

43. Gold, M., Sparer, M., & Chu, K. (1996).

44. Ellwood, P. M., & Lundberg, G. D. (1996). Managed care: A work in progress. *JAMA*, 276 (October 2), 1083-1086.

45. Torrens, P. R. (1988). Historical evolution and overview of health services in the United States. In S. J. Williams & P. R. Torrens (Eds.), *Introduction to Health Services* (pp. 3-31). New York: John Wiley & Sons, p. 8.

46. The Kaiser Commission on the Future of Medicaid (1995). *Medicaid in transition*. Washington, DC: The Henry J. Kaiser Family Foundation.

47. GAO. (1996). *Medicaid managed care: Serving the disabled challenges state programs*, (Report No. GAO/HEHS-96-136). Washington, DC: US Government Printing Office.

48. Kronick, R., Dreyfus, T. (1998). The challenge of risk adjustment for people with disabilities: Health-based payment for Medicaid health plans. *News and Strategies for Managed Medicare & Medicaid*, 4 (8), 4-6.

49. GAO. (1996).

50. Sparer, M. S. (1996).

51. Douglass, R. L., & Torres, R. E. (1994).

52. Wood, D., Halfron, N., Sherbourne, C., & Grabowsky, M. (1994).

53. Showstack, J., Lurie, N., Leatherman, S., Fisher, E., & Inui, T. (1996). Health of the public: Private sector challenge. *JAMA*, 276 (October 2), p. 1072.

54. Lipson, J. (1997). Medicaid managed care and community providers: New partnerships. *Health Affairs*, 16 (4), p. 95.

55. Fisher, I. (1998, February 26).

56. Sparer, M. S. (1996).

57. Gabow, P. (1997). Denver health: Initiatives for survival. *Health Affairs*, 16 (4), 24-26.

58. *Crain's Health Pulse*. (1998, March 23). Managed Care Innovations signs Green Springs. New York: Crain's New York Business.

59. Tobias, C. (1997). *Managed care for special populations: Developing responsive provider networks*. Princeton, NJ: Center for Health Care Strategies, Inc.

60. Lipson, J. (1997).

61. Ibid.

62. Ibid.

63. Goldstein, A. (1998, January 3).

64. Lipson, J. (1997).

65. Dallek, G. (1996). A consumer advocate on Medicaid managed care. *Health Affairs*, 15 (3), 174-177.

66. Holohan, J., Coughlin, T., Ku, L., Lipson, D. J., & Rajan, S. (1995).

67. Ibid.

68. Gold, M., Sparer, M., & Chu, K. (1996), p. 163.

69. Sparer, M. S. (1996).

70. Rosenthal, E. (1996, May 24). Mayor's stalled plans leave public hospitals in trauma. *The New York Times*, p. 1.

71. *Crain's Health Pulse*. (1997, July 16). HHC gets $500 million in waiver. New York: Crain's New York Business.

72. Kaplan, T. (1995). *Health care coverage effects of the Wisconsin welfare reform proposal*. Madison, WI: Institute for Research on Poverty.

73. Wiseman, M. (1996). State strategies for welfare reform: The Wisconsin story. *Journal of Policy Analysis and Management*, 15 (4), 515-545.

74. Gueron, J. M. (1996). A research context for welfare reform. *Journal of Policy Analysis and Management*, 15 (4), 547-561.

75. Pavetti, L. A. (1996, May 23). *Time on welfare and welfare dependency*. (Testimony presented to the House of Representatives Committee

on Ways and Means Subcommittee on Human Resources, 104th Congress). Washington, DC: Urban Institute.

76. Ibid, p. 2.

77. Moffitt, R., & Wolfe, B. (1992). The effect of the Medicaid program on welfare participation and labor supply. *The Review of Economics and Statistics*, 74, 615-626.

78. Quint, J., Bos, J., & Polit, D. (1997). *New Chance: Final Report on a Comprehensive Program for Young Mothers in Poverty and Their Children*. New York: Manpower Demonstration Research Corporation.

CHAPTER 8

Final Thoughts on Conducting Health Care Studies of Homeless Families

This research is unique in examining the health care utilization of families several years after using shelter, and comparing it to that of other poor families who never used shelter. The intent was to paint a clearer picture of how residential instability is—and is not—related to health care use among poor families. The extent to which this was accomplished is subject to the limitations and strengths of the study, discussed below. This chapter concludes with "Final Thoughts" on the contributions of this research to future studies on poor families and their use of primary health care services.

SAMPLING BIAS

Unlike most studies on homeless families, this one sampled only first time shelter users, which eliminated a sampling bias towards long-term shelter users. By contrast, the sample, as a whole, presents a bias towards long-term welfare recipients, as discussed earlier, which may not reflect "typical" welfare recipients. Because New York City's welfare data base was the dominant resource used to relocate families, this sampling bias may have even been greater at follow up than it was at baseline; those no longer on welfare were more difficult to locate.

Because maternal age—being a young mother—is itself a predictor of family homelessness, the comparison sample of never-sheltered families is significantly older than the target sample. Age, in fact, appears to account for the higher degree of poor health among never-sheltered mothers. With age well-established in the literature as a predictor of homelessness, future studies on the effects of homelessness among families would produce a more valid comparison group by matching target and comparison respondents by age. Because the racial/ethnic distribution of homeless families varied significantly from housed, poor mothers, matching by race/ethnicity is an appropriate research strategy as well.

SPECIFICITY OF UTILIZATION OUTCOMES

The outcome measures limit the study's conclusions to general health care use because we measured total annual medical visits, rather than distinguishing by their nature, such as preventive, follow up, sick care or injury. Visits were significantly associated with health status and the number of chronic conditions reported, suggesting that it was a good measure of sick-care utilization, but not necessarily preventive care or other specific types of health care use. Due to this limitation in the specificity of the visit measures, we cannot conclude that prior shelter use is unrelated to the utilization of preventive care or other types of care. Likewise, we cannot rule out that specific aspects of the shelter experience, such as the length of stay, are unrelated to preventive care use. Because there is evidence that homeless families tend to under-utilize preventive care when they reside in shelter, more longitudinal studies on homeless families are needed to focus specifically on families' use of preventive care after homelessness.

Mothers were asked about their regular and most recent source of care, but not how many visits they made to any particular source or for what purpose. Another approach would have been to define a patient's usual source of care as the provider who delivers more than half of the face-to-face ambulatory visits during the year; those without a provider who delivers at least half would be considered not to have a regular source of care.[1] It is impossible to determine from this research to what extent families use multiple sources of care to meet different health care needs.

LIMITATIONS OF THE MODEL

As described earlier, the Behavioral Model of Health Services Use has often been faulted for its low predictability power. The utilization models in this research also showed a similarly weak explanatory power, which could be expected in a study, such as this, for which an individual rather than a geographical entity is the unit of analysis.

Beyond the model itself, the lack of some specific variables may have further reduced its explanatory power.[2,3] Families' health insurance coverage and income, important factors related to health care utilization in general population studies,[4,5] were not explicitly measured in this study. Because the research is a follow-up study of mothers initially on welfare, and most—78 percent—remain on welfare, income is generally very low. Fourteen percent of mothers interviewed at follow up were earning incomes below poverty, despite being off welfare, leaving only 8 percent who were off welfare and earning incomes above the poverty level. Given that employment is also extremely low (11% of the sample), and given the job opportunities available, very few mothers are likely to have been covered by private health insurance.

Public assistance status, a significant enabling factor associated with families' use of health care, served as a proxy for having access to Medicaid, most likely the only kind of health coverage that was available to this sample of mothers. With welfare reform and expansions of state health insurance programs for children underway, future longitudinal studies on poor families may require more specificity about the types of insurance coverage and benefits available to individual family members, and may need to account for periods of non-coverage among family members.

Excluded altogether from the conceptual model was the notion of health beliefs. Andersen and Newman assert that attitudes and beliefs about disease and the health care system, namely physicians, indirectly influence utilization behavior.[6] However, Wolinskly reports that Berkanovic and colleagues conducted several studies showing that only health beliefs about a particular disease predicted behavior related to that disease; general health beliefs did not predict general utilization outcomes.[7] Since this study only included general outcomes—unrelated to a specific illness—the exclusion of health beliefs most likely did not produce a significant loss in explained variance.

DATA COLLECTION

The use of self-reported or institutional data can produce multiple threats to internal validity,[8] some of which apply to this study. Recall problems are an overriding issue, since almost all of the data were self-reported. The most serious errors in responses are likely to have occurred with quantitative questions, particularly those pertaining to a year's time or a longer period, as has been documented elsewhere.[9,10]

It is impossible to determine whether overall differences in housing experiences between ever-sheltered and never-sheltered families may have biased either group to understate or overstate their mobility or length of stay in any one place, or even their reporting on medical visits, but such biases may exist. Gelberg and Siecke, in summarizing research on homeless adults' self-reports, found that they were fairly accurate in reporting whether they had made a medical visit in a given time period, but were less accurate than those surveyed in general population studies.[11]

Family-type surveys, such as this one, require a mother to report on items for each of her children as well as herself. Questions, such as the number of medical visits in the last year, have been found to produce more conservative answers among larger families.[12] Respondent recall problems may explain the more conservative responses; fatigue and loss of motivation for those who must give more responses may also contribute to the differences. This potential problem was limited by soliciting information about no more than one child from each of four different age groups. Mothers typically reported on one or two children.

Social desirability most likely affected reporting on health problems, particularly stigmatized conditions such as HIV/AIDS, as well as mental health problems and substance abuse or treatment. However, Gelberg and Siecke report on several studies of homeless adults that showed how the effects of social desirability on sensitive questions could be mitigated by providing a non-threatening environment and establishing a rapport with respondents through ethnic and gender matching.[13] We attempted to overcome social desirability effects by matching interviewers with respondents, based on language and gender, and by allowing respondents to choose between being interviewed at home or in our offices. To the extent respondents underreported on stigmatized conditions or events, we could expect social desirability to affect ever-sheltered and never-sheltered responses equally.

The potential "longitudinal" benefits of this study were impeded by a lack of data on mothers' utilization at baseline. The Medicaid baseline data on emergency department use showed significant differences by shelter status prior to Time 1, but was available only for a limited number of mothers. Conclusions about mothers' utilization patterns prior to shelter use are impossible to make without having actually measured respondents' health care utilization at Time 1. Such data were not collected because the initial study focused on the predictors of homelessness and not health care use in particular.

GENERALIZATION OF FINDINGS

Overall, the results of this research are best generalized to sheltered and never-sheltered long-term welfare recipients in New York City. Despite differences in sampling strategies, the characteristics of families in this study are similar, respectively, to those found in studies of homeless and housed poor families conducted elsewhere. It is likely that formerly homeless families in other urban localities also have a higher relative risk of using public and hospital-based sources of health care, to the extent they are available in their communities. Other significant findings from the analyses may or may not be suitable for generalizing to long-term welfare recipients from other large, urban areas. Differences in welfare benefits and restrictions across states, and homeless shelter policies across cities may limit the extent to which generalizations can extend beyond New York City.

The policy recommendations regarding formerly homeless families and managed care are based on research conducted within New York's unique political and policy environment, in which a right to shelter, historically, has been unconditionally provided to city residents. The general concept of connecting formerly homeless families with appropriate managed care health plans seems applicable to other urban cities, but likely depends on the sophistication of the existing public and/or private infrastructure that serves homeless families, among other factors. Unclear, is the level of residential stability that families achieve after leaving homeless shelters in localities with different shelter policies and subsidized housing programs. Even less understood is the degree to which formerly homeless families on Medicaid may have different experiences under managed care than never-sheltered Medicaid families. Future studies should address this area, particularly with the trend towards mandatory Medicaid managed care.

The generalization of findings applies to the period of the late 1980s through the early 1990s. Since families were first sampled in

1988, the profile of homeless families in New York City has been changing to one of younger, less independent and larger families.[14] In addition, federal support for low income housing is at an all-time low; predictably, so is the availability of decent, low-income housing in New York City and around the country.[15,16] The findings of this study may, in fact, understate the existing relationship between a tenuous housing history and a tenuous connection with the health care system. Should time limits on shelter stays or a fixed reimbursement system (a managed care approach) replace the current per diem payment system in New York, the role of the family shelter system as a gateway to obtaining permanent housing could diminish as well.[17]

FINAL THOUGHTS

Research that helps us understand, more precisely, the dynamics of poor families' experiences with residential instability can play an important role in identifying the type of support families need, and when, and may help generate policy innovations to meet those needs. This study represents one example of research in this direction. It also highlights the need for more longitudinal studies on the dynamics of family homelessness in an environment of dynamic welfare, health care and housing policies.

By theoretically including residential mobility in their original Behavioral Model of Health Services Use, Andersen and Newman tacitly acknowledged residential instability as a factor in health care utilization.[18] In practice, residential instability is largely ignored in health services research. Despite the models' overall low predictive power, the research demonstrated the important role of residential instability regarding where poor families seek health care. Regardless of the analytical model used, future health care utilization studies on poor families are likely to benefit from including a measure of residential instability. The simple question, "Have you ever lived in a homeless shelter?" may be a practical way to measure it. The answer is likely to be a strong predictor of where poor families currently seek healthcare. That is, until we have policies that empower formerly homeless families to connect with mainstream health care providers, and we require those providers to be more accountable to the health care needs of *all* poor families.

NOTES

1. Weiner, J. P., Starfield, B. H., Powe, N. R., Stuart, M. E., & Steinwachs, D. M. (1996). Ambulatory care practice variation within a Medicaid program. *Health Services Research*, 30 (6), 751-769.

2. Mohr, L. B. (1988). *Impact analysis for program evaluation*. Chicago: The Dorsey Press.

3. Judd, C. M., & Kenny, D. A. (1981). *Estimating the effects of social interventions*. Cambridge, MA: Cambridge University Press.

4. Freeman, H. E., Blendon, R. J., Aiken, L. H., Sudman, S., Mullinix, C. F., & Corey, C. R. (1987). Americans report on their access to health care. *Health Affairs*, 6 (1), 7-15.

5. Mechanic, D., & Aiken, L. (1989). Chapter 9: Access to health care and use of medical care services. In H. E. Freeman, & S. Levine (Eds.), *Handbook of Medical Sociology* (4th ed., pp. 166-242), Englewood Cliffs, NJ: Prentice Hall.

6. Andersen, R. M., & Newman, J. F. (1973). Societal and individual determinants of medical care utilization in the United States. *The Milbank Memorial Fund Quarterly*, 51(1), 95-121.

7. Wolinsky, F. D. (1978). Assessing the effects of predisposing, enabling and illness-morbidity characteristics on health service utilization. *Journal of Health and Social Behavior*, 19, 384-396.

8. Nachmias, D., & Nachmias, C. (1981). *Research methods in the social sciences*. New York: St. Martin's Press.

9. Groves, R. M. (1989). *Survey errors and survey costs*. New York: John Wiley & Sons.

10. Cannell, C., Miller P., Oksenber, L. (1981). Research on interviewing techniques. In: S. Leinhardt (ed.), *Sociological Methodology*. San Francisco: Jossey-Bass Publishers.

11. Gelberg, L., & Siecke, N. (1997). Accuracy of homeless adults' self-reports. *Medical Care*, 35 (3), 287-290.

12. Litman, T. J. (1974). The family as a basic unit in health and medical care: A social behavioral overview. *Social Science Medicine*, 8, 495-519.

13. Gelberg, L., & Siecke, N. (1997).

14. Homes for the Homeless. (1992, June). A generation of homeless families. *The New Poverty*, pp. 17.

15. DeParle, J. (1996, October 20). Slamming the door. *The New York Times Magazine*, pp. 52-63.

16. Kennedy, R. (1998, March 4). Availability of rent aid is reduced. *The New York Times*, p. B1, B6.

17. Culhane, D. P., & Wachter, S. (1996, June). *Homelessness and public shelter provision in New York City*. Paper presented at the annual meeting of Health Care for the Homeless, Washington, DC.

18. Andersen, R. M., & Newman, J. F. (1973).

APPENDIX A

The New York City Family Shelter System

The following overview of the policies and procedures that guided the lives of those who became part of the New York City Family Shelter System in the late 1980s through early 1990s is provided as contextual background on the homeless families of this study. Most cities do not have a distinct bureaucracy to regulate or manage homeless families. New York has separate shelter systems that do both for homeless families and single adults. As discussed below, certain policies may have influenced the composition of families entering the shelter system, as well as the length of stay of their homelessness and the quality of their shelter experience.

Three New York City court cases, in 1981, 1983 and 1986, made access to shelter a right for any family or person seeking it.[1] Most families entering shelter are receiving some form of public assistance. In addition, a household of two or more individuals on either Home Relief assistance (for adults with no child custody), Emergency Assistance to Needy Families with Children, Emergency Assistance to Aged, Blind and Disabled Persons, or Supplemental Security Income may also become clients of the shelter system.[2] Families not on public assistance may apply for it when they first seek emergency housing.

Until 1989, a family could be referred to one, two or all three types of shelter: 1) Barracks or congregate-style facilities, called Tier I; 2) "Welfare" hotels/motels; and 3) apartment-style family centers and shelters, called Tier II. Beginning in 1989, specialized shelters for childless couples and pregnant women were created.[3,4] By 1992, three specialized facilities were serving 11 percent of homeless families.

New York City's homeless policies during the late 1980s allowed families who became homeless, for any other reason than a fire or vacate order, to request shelter at one of four emergency assistance units (EAUs) operated by the city's welfare agency, the Human Resources Administration.[5] Families affected by fire or evictions were allowed a direct route to Tier II housing and speedier access to re-housing. All families had a right to emergency housing located as near as possible to their children's school and their former community.

The four Tier I facilities located in each borough, except Staten Island, served as receiving centers for homeless families. From 1987 to 1991, the monthly average number of families staying at least one night in a Tier I shelter slowly climbed from 476 to 497. By fiscal year (FY) 1992, the average had dropped to 198.[6] At a minimum, Tier I shelters were required to provide "a sleeping area, access to three nutritional meals a day, supervision, a preliminary needs determination and health services."[7] Families were limited to 21-day stays in Tier I shelters, after which time, the city was required to transfer them to a hotel or Tier II shelter. Families could be exempted from a Tier I shelter placement if a family member was pregnant, was a newborn child under six months, had a contagious disease, or had medical or psychological needs that could not be met in a Tier I shelter. If a family remained in a Tier I facility after such time, it was entitled to receive the same services offered at Tier II facilities. Some have argued that the higher standards for pregnant women, and their more favorable placement in the queue for permanent housing, created an incentive for pregnant women to seek shelter.

Until the expansion of Tier II family shelters, most families spent their longest time in temporary housing at commercially operated "welfare" hotels and motels. In FY 1987, 3300, or about 72 percent of homeless families were housed in a welfare hotel.[8] State regulations for standards of care and services generally included providing "safe conditions," baby formula and diet-necessary foods (or a restaurant allowance), access to refrigeration for medications, laundry facilities and pay phones.[9] By all accounts, welfare hotels were the least compliant towards meeting these standards.[10] Hotel operators had full discretion to limit a family's stay to a maximum of 28 days, or to allow an indefinite stay until a family found another arrangement.[11] After 30 days, a family is entitled to tenancy status, under New York law. Hotel management was required to follow city and state statutes in order to evict a family from its premises legally.

The services provided to homeless families living in hotels varied widely. At a minimum, all reportedly were visited periodically by public health nurses who provided health assessments, education, referrals and follow-up as part of the city health department's Homeless Health Initiative.[12] At some hotels, additional health services were made available through arrangements with and referrals to neighborhood providers. Typical affiliations included nearby public hospitals or medical centers, community health and mental health clinics, child health stations and family planning centers. In some cases, nurses or physicians made weekly visits to a shelter. How well these practices were followed remains unclear.

The lack of amenities and abundance of squalor, for which the welfare hotels were notorious,[13] eventually prompted the city to reduce its reliance on hotels and increase the supply of Tier II family shelters. Tier II shelters, which remain in operation today, were created, in part, to assist families with finding and preparing for permanent housing. Service requirements include access to services provided at Tier I facilities, except that families stay in apartment-style private units. Tier II facilities are also required to provide recreational services, and information and referral services for child care.[14]

Tier II shelters are operated by not-for-profit organizations which are reimbursed by the City on a per diem family rate.[15] Less than 20 percent of New York City's homeless families were housed in Tier II shelters in 1987 because there were so few in operation. There were 57 hotels and 17 family shelters in operation at that time. By 1992, a complete switch had occurred, with 60 Tier II family shelters and only 20 commercial hotels in use.[16] A family residing in a Tier II shelter faces no maximum stay. However, after a family has resided in shelter for 12 months or longer, HRA is required to offer the family a permanent place to live. HRA is to arrange for the family to visit several apartments and choose among them. The agency also reimburses families for moving expenses.

From 1989 to 1991, 4072 families, on average, were provided permanent housing each year. In this same three-year period, 59 percent of families, on average, (including some individuals) were relocated to apartments owned by the City's Housing Preservation Department (HPD).[17] HPD apartments are those confiscated from owners who have reneged on their property taxes or have failed to maintain the property. Another 31 percent of homeless families, on average, were re-housed in one of the City's public housing project apartment buildings. About 10 percent of families were housed in an apartment through the Emergency Assistance Re-housing Program (EARP), which subsidizes private owners to provide apartments to formerly homeless families.

NOTES

1. Women's City Club of New York. (1992). *Beyond Facilities and Good Intentions*, New York: The Coalition for the Homeless.
2. Department of Social Services. (1988). Programs for homeless children and families. *Homelessness performance report*, Albany, NY: State of New York.
3. Mayor's Office on Homelessness and SRO Housing for the City of New York. (1992). *Fact Sheet: Homelessness in New York City*. New York: City of New York.
4. Department of City Planning. (1992). *Annual report on social indicators*. New York: City of New York.
5. Coalition for the Homeless. (1989). *Reference manual for food, shelter and resources for the homeless*. New York: Coalition for the Homeless.
6. Department of City Planning. (1992).
7. Department of Social Services. (1988), p. 159.
8. Mayor's Office on Homelessness and SRO Housing for the City of New York. (1992).
9. Coalition for the Homeless. (1989), p. 126.
10. Women's City Club of New York. (1992).
11. Human Resources Administration. (1990). *Fact Sheets*. New York: City of New York, Division of Adult Services Administration.
12. Ibid.
13. Bach, V., & Steinhagen, R. (1987). *Alternatives to the welfare hotel: Using emergency assistance to provide decent transitional shelter for homeless families*. New York: Community Service Society of New York.
14. Department of Social Services. (1988).
15. Ibid.
16. Mayor's Office on Homelessness and SRO Housing for the City of New York. (1992).

17. Housing Preservation and Development. (1991). *Housing and vacancy report: New York City 1991* (Source: U.S. Bureau of the Census Housing and Vacancy Report). New York: City of New York.

APPENDIX B

Predictors of Being Interviewed at Follow Up

This research was based on a sample of families who were part of a follow up study of 838 families originally interviewed in 1988. Excluding the deceased, odds ratios were calculated to determine what characteristics, if any, predicted being interviewed at Time 2 (Table B.1). The most significant predictor of being interviewed was the amount of time that interviewers spent in the field searching for a respondent. In other words, persistence paid off. Those re-interviewed at follow up were less likely to be one of a small group of other ethnic backgrounds (white, Native American, Asian). Mothers who spent any time in the single adult shelter system after their Time 1 interview were also less likely to be re-interviewed.

The only other strong predictor of being interviewed at Time 2 appears to be an anomaly. Mothers who reported two or more problems with the building they were living in, during the year before their Time 1 interview, were twice as likely to be re-interviewed as those with less than two building problems. Building problems included living in a place with rodents; with no heat or running water for a week at a time or more; or which was closed, condemned, or was unsafe because of drugs or crime.

Characteristics related to personal problems, such as using rehabilitation services for substance abuse, serving time in jail, or having an overnight stay in a mental hospital, as reported by respondents at Time 1, were not significant predictors of being interviewed, nor were traumatic childhood experiences related to family separation, a history of domestic violence, or giving birth before age 18.

Table B.1: Adjusted Odds Ratios of Being Interviewed at Follow-up

Characteristics at Time 1, unless Otherwise Noted	Eligible for Follow-up Sample (N=819)[a]
	Odds Ratio (95% CI)[b]
Nº. Months in Field, 1992-1993	1.2 (1.1, 1.2)**
Living Situation	
Requested Shelter *(base is housed)*	1.1 (0.7, 1.6)
In Single Adult Shelter Anytime between 1988-1993	0.5 (0.2, 1.0)*
Address Outside of NYC	0.6 (0.3, 1.1)
Nº. Places Lived in Last 3 Years	1.0 (0.8, 1.1)
2 or More Building Problems	2.2 (1.5, 3.1)**
Demographics	
Age 30 or Older	1.0 (0.7, 1.5)
Race/Ethnicity *(base is Latina)*	
Black	0.9 (0.6, 1.4)
Other	0.4 (0.2, 0.7)**
Marital Status *(base is Married)*	
Single, Divorced, Other	0.7 (0.4, 1.1)
High School Diploma/ GED	1.0 (0.7, 1.4)
Ever Worked Full or Part-time	0.9 (0.7, 1.3)
Experienced Childhood Poverty	0.7 (0.5, 1.1)
Experienced Teen Pregnancy	0.9 (0.6, 1.4)
Personal Problems before Time 1	
Alcohol or Drug Rehab	0.9 (0.3, 2.3)
Jail/Prison	1.3 (0.4, 4.4)
Mental Hospitalization	1.2 (0.3, 3.8)
Health Problem	1.0 (0.6, 1.5)
Family Separation before 18	
Experienced any of the following:	1.1 (0.7, 1.7)
Foster Home	
Institution/group Home	
Ran Away	
Lived on the Streets	
Sexually Abused	
Physically Abused	

[a] Includes mothers eligible for Time 2 study; excludes deceased mothers.
[b] Confidence Interval
*P<.05; ** P<.01

APPENDIX C

A Note on the Use of Multinomial Logistic Regression

For the dependent variable related to regular source of health care, mothers could give any one of a number of possible answers about where they and their children usually go for care when they are sick or need advice about health matters. Thus, the dependent variable has multiple categories, which makes multinomial logistic regression (MLR) an appropriate technique to use in conducting analyses on regular source of care.[1]

RELATIVE RISK RATIOS

Results for analyses on source of care outcomes are presented as relative risk ratios (RRR). Using the simple tabulation of source of care responses among mothers, shown in the table below, an example of how to compute and interpret relative risk ratios is presented, based on an explanation by Hamilton and Seyfrit.[2]

Table C.1: Tabulations of Mothers' Regular Source of Care

Source of Care	Ever-Sheltered	Never-Sheltered	Total
Doc/HMO	58	156	214
HospOPD	79	80	159
CommClinic	55	32	87
ER/NoReg	56	22	78
Total	248	290	538

Table C.2: Stata MLR Output for Mothers' Source of Care

```
Multinomial regression                        Number of obs =      538
                                              chi2(3)       =    64.80
                                              Prob > chi2   =   0.0000

Log Likelihood = -667.83455
------------------------------------------------------------------------
Source   |    RRR    Std. Err.       z      P>|z|      [95% Conf. Interval]
---------+--------------------------------------------------------------
HospOPD  |
evershlt| 2.65603  0.586796    4.421   0.000       1.72257     4.09533
---------+--------------------------------------------------------------
PubClin  |
evershlt| 4.62284  1.24973     5.663   0.000       2.72142     7.85276
---------+--------------------------------------------------------------
ER/NoReg|
evershlt| 6.84639  2.01896     6.523   0.000       3.84103    12.20327
---------+--------------------------------------------------------------
(Outcome Source==Doc/HMO is the comparison group)
```

Note that because less than 2 percent of all mothers reported a source of care other than one of the four major categories shown in Table C.1, the responses from the "other" category were excluded from these analyses.

For this example, the "ED/No regular source of care" category was selected for comparison to a reference category, namely, the category of private doctor/HMO. Among ever-sheltered mothers, the ratio of using an ED/No regular source of care over a private doctor/HMO is: P (Use ED/No reg source) ÷ P (Use Doctor/HMO) = (56/248) ÷ (58/248) = 0.96551. Among never-sheltered mothers, the ratio of using an ED/No Regular Source over a private doctor/HMO is: P (Use ED/No reg source) ÷ P (Use Doctor/HMO) = (22/290) ÷ (156/290) = 0.14102.

The ratio of these two ratios (0.96551 ÷ 0.14102) equals the relative risk ratio (RRR = 6.84639) displayed in the last row of the MLR results obtained from using Stata statistical software (Table C.2). The results show that the relative risk of using an ED/No Regular Source over a private doctor/HMO as a regular source of care is almost seven times higher for ever-sheltered mothers than it is for never-sheltered mothers. Note that the output gives the reference or comparison category for source of care as "Doc/HMO," from which the RRR's for other categories are compared as well.

NOTES

1. Homer, D Jr., & Lemeshow, S. (1989). *Applied Logistic Regression.* New York: John Wiley & Sons.

2. Hamilton, L. C., & Seyfrit, C. L. (1993, May). Interpreting multinomial logistic regression. *Stata Technical Bulletin.* Santa Monica, CA: Computing Resource Center.

Bibliography

Aday, L. A. (1993). Indicators and predictors of health services utilization. In S. J. Williams, & P. R. Torrens (Eds.), *Introduction to Health Services* (4th ed., pp. 46-70). Albany, NY: Delmar Publishing, Inc.

Alperstein, G., Rappaport, C., & Flanigan, J. M. (1988). Health problems of homeless children in New York City. *American Journal of Public Health*, 78 (9), 1232-1233.

American Hospital Association. (1994). *Guide to the Health Care Field.* Chicago, IL: Author.

Andersen, R. M. (1995). Revisiting the behavioral model and access to medical care: Does it matter? *Journal of Health and Social Behavior*, 36, 1-10.

Andersen, R. M., Aday, L. A., & Chen, M. S. (1986). Health status and health care utilization. *Health Affairs*, 5 (1), 154-169.

Andersen, R. M., & Newman, J. F. (1973). Societal and individual determinants of medical care utilization in the United States. *The Milbank Memorial Fund Quarterly*, 51(1), 95-121.

Angus, D. C., Linde-Swirble, W. T., Sirio, C. A., Rotondi, A. J., Chelluri, L., Newbold, R. C., Lave, J. R., & Pinsky, M. R. (1996). The effect of managed care on ICU length of stay. *JAMA*, 276 (October 2), 1075-1082.

Ashworth, K., Hill, M., & Walker, R. (1994). Patterns of childhood poverty: New challenges for policy. *Journal of Policy Analysis and Management*, 13 (4), 658-680.

Bach, V., & Steinhagen, R. (1987). *Alternatives to the welfare hotel: Using emergency assistance to provide decent transitional shelter for homeless families*. New York: Community Service Society of New York.

Bane, M. J., & Ellwood, D. T. (1986). Slipping into and out of poverty: The dynamics of spells. *Inquiry*, 21 (Winter), 1-23.

Banta, H. D. (1990). What is health care? In A. R. Kovner (Ed.), *Health care delivery in the United States* (4th ed., pp. 8-30), New York: Springer Publishing Company.

Bashshur, R. L., Homan, R. K., & Smith, D. G. (1994). Beyond the uninsured: Problems in access to care. *Medical Care*, 32 (5), 409-419.

Bass, J. L., Brennan, P., Mehta, K., & Kodzis, S. (1990). Pediatric problems in a suburban shelter for homeless families. *Pediatrics*, 85 (1), 33-38.

Bassuk, E. L. (1991). Homeless families. *Scientific American*, 265 (December), 66-74.

Bassuk, E. L., Buckner, J. C., Weinreb, L. F., Browne, A., Bassuk, S. S., Dawson, R., Perloff, J. N. (1997). Homelessness in female-headed families: Childhood and adult risk and protective factors. *American Journal of Public Health*, 87 (2), 241-248.

Bassuk, E. L., & Rosenberg, L. (1990). Psychosocial characteristics of homeless children and children with homes. *Pediatrics*, 85 (3), 257-261.

Bassuk, E. L., Rubin, L., & Lauriat, A. S. (1986). Characteristics of sheltered homeless families. *American Journal of Public Health*, 76 (9), 1097-1101.

Bassuk, E. L., Weinreb, L. F., Buckner, J. C., Browne, A., Salomon, A., & Bassuk, S. S. (1996). The characteristics and needs of sheltered homeless and low-income housed mothers. *JAMA*, 276 (August 28), 640-646.

Baxter, R. J., & Mechanic, R. E. (1997). The status of local health care safety nets. *Health Affairs*, 16 (4), 7-23.

Bazzoli, G. J. (1986). Health care for the indigent: Overview of critical issues. *Health Services Research*, 21(3), 353-402.

Berkanovic, E., & Reeder, L. G. (1974). Can money buy the appropriate use of services? Some notes on the meaning of utilization data. *Journal of Health & Social Behavior*, 15 (June), 93-99.

Berlin, G., & McAllister, W. (1994). Homeless family shelters and family homelessness. *American Behavioral Scientist*, 37 (3), 422-434.

Berry, C. A., & Weitzman, B. C. (1993). Factors affecting housing comfort among formerly homeless families: Housing quality or individual vulnerabilities? *The Community Psychologist*, 26 (Spring), 27-29.

Billings, J., Zeitel, L., Lukomnik, J., Carey, T. S., Blank, A. E., & Newman, L. (1993). Impact of socioeconomic status on hospital use in New York City. *Health Affairs*, 12, 162-173.

Bloom, B. (1995). Health insurance and medical care: Health of our nation's children, United States, 1988. *Advance data from vital and health statistics*, (series 16, No. 19). Washington, DC: National Center for Health Statistics.

Blumberg, L.J., & Liska, D. W. (1996). *The uninsured in the United States: A status report*. Washington, DC: The Urban Institute.

Bodenheimer, T. S., & Grumbach, K. (1996). Capitation or decapitation. *JAMA*, 276 (October 2), 1025-1031.

Braveman, P., Bennett, T., Lewis, C., Egerter, S., & Showstack, J. (1993,). Access to prenatal care following major Medicaid eligibility expansions. *JAMA*, 269 (March 10), 1285-1289.

Brickner, P. W., Scharer-Keen L., Conanan, B., Elvy, A., & Savarese, M. (1985). *Health care of homeless people*. New York: Springer Publishing Company.

Burg, M. A. (1994). Health problems of sheltered homeless women and their dependent children. *Health & Social Work*, 19 (2), 125-131.

Burt, M. R. (1992). *Over the edge: The growth of homelessness in the 1980s*. New York: Russell Sage Foundation.

Burt, M., & Cohen, B. (1989). Differences among homeless single women, women with children and single men. *Social Problems*, 35 (5), 508-524.

Cannell, C., Miller P., Oksenber, L. (1981). Research on interviewing techniques. In: S. Leinhardt (ed.), *Sociological Methodology*. San Francisco, CA: Jossey-Bass Publishers.

Carr, W., Cohen, S., Schop, J. A., & Rink, R. (1988). An unfinished agenda: Reducing the health deficit. In M. I. Krasner (Ed.), *Poverty and health in New York City* (pp. 21-47). New York: United Hospital Fund.

Chavkin, W., Kristal, A., Seabron, C., & Guigli, P. E. (1987). Reproductive experiences of women living in hotels for the homeless in New York City. *New York State Journal of Medicine*, 87, 10-13.

Clancy, C., Cooper, J., & Leopold, N. (1996). Sustained partnerships in primary care. *The Journal of Family Practice*, 42 (2), 129-137.

Coalition for the Homeless. (1989). *Reference manual for food, shelter and resources for the homeless*. New York: Coalition for the Homeless.

Community Service Society of New York (1990). Home relief. In Starr (Ed.), *The intensive case management resource on entitlements and services*. New York: City University of New York, Hunter College, Department of Social Services.

Cornelius, L J. (1997). The degree of usual provider continuity for African and Latino Americans. *Journal of Health Care for the Poor and Underserved*, 8 (2), 170-185.

Counte, M. A., & Christman, L. P. (1981). *Interpersonal behavior and health care*. Boulder, CO: Westview Press.

Cousineau, M. R., Wittenberg, E., & Pollatsek, J. (1995). *A study of the health care for the homeless program*. Report to U.S. Department of Health and Human Services, Public Health Service, Health Resources and Services Administration, Bureau of Primary Health Care, Special Populations Division.

Cowal, K., Shinn, M., & Stojanovic, D. (1996, October). *Parent-child separations among homeless and poor housed families in New York City*. Paper presented at the annual meeting of the American Public Health Association, New York, NY.

Crain's Health Pulse. (1997, July 16). HHC gets $500 million in waiver. New York: Crain's New York Business.

Crain's Health Pulse. (1998, March 23). Managed Care Innovations signs Green Springs. New York: Crain's New York Business.

Culhane, D. P., Dejowski, E. F., Ibanez, J., Needham, E., & Macchia, I. (1993). *Public Shelter Admission Rates in Philadelphia and New York City*. Washington, DC: Office of Housing Research, Fannie Mae.

Culhane, D. P., & Wachter, S. (1996, June). *Homelessness and public shelter provision in New York City*. Paper presented at the annual meeting of Health Care for the Homeless, Washington, DC.

Cunningham, P. J., & Cornelius, L. J. (1995). Access to ambulatory care for American Indians and Alaska natives: The relative importance of personal and community resources. *Social Science Medicine*, 40 (3), 393-407.

Cutts, D.B., Pheley, A.M., & Geppert, J.S. (1996, October). *Profile of young children with a history of homelessness receiving care at an inner-city hospital clinic*. Paper presented at the meeting of the American Public Health Association, New York, NY.

Dallek, G. (1996). A consumer advocate on Medicaid managed care. *Health Affairs*, 15 (3), 174-177.

Davis, K., & Rowland, D. (1991). Financing health care for the poor. In E. Ginzberg (Ed.), *Health Services Research* (pp. 93-125). Cambridge, MA: Harvard University Press, 93-125.

DeParle, J. (1996, October 20). Slamming the door. *The New York Times Magazine*, pp. 52-63.

DeParle, J. (1997, December 30). Success, and frustration, as welfare rules change. *The New York Times*, pp. 1, 16, 17.

Department of City Planning. (1992). *Annual report on social indicators*. New York: City of New York.

Department of Homeless Services. (1998). *Services at the department of homeless services*, [website: www.ci.nyc.us/html/dhs/html/dhsserv.html] p. 2, New York: City of New York.

Dornbusch, S. M. (1994). Additional perspectives on homeless families. *American Behavioral Scientist*, 37 (3), 404-411.

Douglass, R. L., & Torres, R. E. (1994). Evaluation of a managed care program for the non-Medicaid urban poor. *Journal of Health Care for the Poor and Underserved*, 5, 83-97.

Dutton, D. B. (1978). Explaining the low use of health services by the poor: Costs, attitudes, or delivery systems? *American Sociological Review*, 43 (6), 348-368.

Duvall, D., & Booth, A. (1978). The housing environment and women's health. *Journal of Health & Social Behavior*, 19 (December), 410-417.

Eckert, J. K., & Goldstein, M. C. (1983). An anthropological approach to the study of illness behavior in an urban community. *Urban Anthropology*, 12 (2), 125-137.

Ell, K., & Northern, H. (1990). *Families and health care*. New York: Aldine de Gruyter.

Ellwood, P. M., & Lundberg, G. D. (1996). Managed care: A work in progress. *JAMA*, 276 (October 2), 1083-1086.

Fantasia, R., & Isserman, M. (1994). *Homelessness: A sourcebook*. New York: Facts on File, Inc.

Fierman, A. H., Dreyer, B. P., Quinn, L., Shulman, S., Courtlandt, C., & Guzzo, R. (1991). Growth delay in homeless children. *Pediatrics*, 88 (5), 918-925.

Finder, A. (1998, April 12). Evidence is scant that workfare leads to full-time jobs. *The New York Times*, pp. 1, 30.

Fine, J., Foltin, G., Tunik, M., Fierman, A., & Dreyer, B. (1990). Ambulance utilization by homeless children. *American Journal of Childhood Diseases*, 144 (April), 433.

Fischer, P. J., & Breakey, W. R. (1991). The epidemiology of alcohol, drug, and mental disorders among homeless persons. *American Psychologist*, 46 (11), 1115-1128.

Fisher, I. (1998, February 26). HMO drops Medicaid in Connecticut. *The New York Times*, pp. 1, 6.

Fowler, M. G., Simpson, G. A., & Schoendorf, K. C. (1993). Families on the move and children's health care. *Pediatrics*, 91 (5), 934-940.

Frederick Schneiders Research (1996). *Medicaid and managed care: Focus group studies of low-income Medicaid beneficiaries in five states* (Report prepared for the Henry J. Kaiser Family Foundation). Washington, DC: Author.

Freeman, H. E., Blendon, R. J., Aiken, L. H., Sudman, S., Mullinix, C. F., & Corey, C. R. (1987). Americans report on their access to health care. *Health Affairs*, 6, 7-15.

Freund, P. E. S., & McGuire, M. B. (1991). *Health, illness, and the social body*. Englewood Cliffs, NJ: Prentice Hall.

Gabow, P. (1997). Denver health: Initiatives for survival. *Health Affairs*, 16 (4), 24-26.

Gelberg, L., Gallagher, T. C., Andersen, R. M., & Koegel, P. (1997). Competing priorities as a barrier to medical care among homeless adults in Los Angeles. *American Journal of Public Health*, 87 (2), 217-220.

Gelberg, L., & Siecke, N. (1997). Accuracy of homeless adults' self-reports. *Medical Care*, 35 (3), 287-290.

General Accounting Office [GAO]. (1995). Uninsured and children on Medicaid (from Report No. GAO/HEHS-95-83R). *Medical Benefits*, 12 (8), 4.

GAO. (1996). *Medicaid managed care: Serving the disabled challenges state programs*, (Report No. GAO/HEHS-96-136). Washington, DC: US Government Printing Office.

GAO. (1997). *Medicaid Managed Care: The challenge of holding plans accountable requires greater state effort*, (Report No. GAO/HEHS-97-86). Washington, DC: US Government Printing Office.

Gold, M., Sparer, M., & Chu, K. (1996). Medicaid managed care: Lessons from five states. *Health Affairs*, 15 (3), 153-165.

Goldman, B. (1993). Improving access to the underserved through Medicaid managed care. *Journal of Health Care for the Poor and Underserved*, 4 (3), 290-308.

Goldstein, A. (1998, January 3). Clinics losing ground in drive toward managed care. *The Washington Post*, pp. 1, 10, 11.

Goodman, L. A. (1991). The relationship between social support and family homelessness: A comparison study of homeless and housed mothers. *Journal of Community Psychology*, 19 (October), 321-332.

Gordon, S. (1996). *Removing barriers, improving choices: A case study on reproductive health services in managed care settings*. New York: Center for Reproductive Law & Policy.

Groves, R. M. (1989). *Survey errors and survey costs*. New York: John Wiley & Sons.

Guendelman, S., & Schwalbe, J. (1986). Medical care utilization by Hispanic children. *Medical Care*, 24 (10), 925-940.

Gueron, J. M., (1996). A research context for welfare reform. *Journal of Policy Analysis and Management*, 15 (4), 547-561.

Hamilton, L. C., & Seyfrit, C. L. (1993, May). Interpreting multinomial logistic regression. *Stata Technical Bulletin.* Santa Monica, CA: Computing Resource Center.

Health Care Finance Administration [HCFA]. (1996). *National summary of Medicaid managed care programs and enrollment as of June 30 of each year.* Baltimore, MD: U.S. Department of Health and Human Services.

HCFA. (1997, August 19). Managed care in Medicare and Medicaid. *Fact Sheet* (website: www. hcfa.gov/facts/f960900.html). Baltimore, MD: US Department of Health and Human Services.

HCFA. (1998, February 28). *National summary of Medicaid managed care programs and enrollment* (website: www.hcfa.gov/medicaid/plansum7 .html). Baltimore, MD: US Department of Health and Human Services.

Heller, P. L., Chalfant, H. P., Quesada, G. M., & Rivera-Worley, M. D. C. (1981). Class, familism and utilization of health services in Durango, Mexico: A replication. *Social Science Medicine*, 15A, 539-541.

Hellinger, F. J. (1996). The expanding scope of state legislation. *JAMA*, 276 (October 2), 1065-1070.

Holloway, L. (1998, February 8). City asks an earlier verdict on shelter eviction rules. *The New York Times*, p. 37.

Holohan, J., Coughlin, T., Ku, L., Lipson, D. J., & Rajan, S. (1995). Insuring the poor through section 1115 Medicaid waivers. *Health Affairs*, 14 (1), 199-216.

Homer, D Jr., & Lemeshow, S. (1989). *Applied Logistic Regression.* New York: John Wiley & Sons.

Homes for the Homeless. (1992). A generation of homeless families. *The New Poverty* (June), pp. 1-7.

Homes for the Homeless. (1997). *Homelessness: The foster care connection.* New York: Institute for Children and Poverty.

Housing Preservation and Development. (1991). *Housing and vacancy report: New York City 1991* (Source: U.S. Bureau of the Census Housing and Vacancy Report). New York: City of New York.

Human Resources Administration. (1990). *Fact Sheets.* New York: City of New York, Division of Adult Services Administration.

Iglehart, J. K. (1995). Health policy report: Medicaid and managed care. *New England Journal of Medicine*, 332 (June 22), 1727-1731.

Ineichen, B. (1993). *Homes and health: How housing and health interact.* London: E & FN.

Institute of Medicine. (1988). *Homelessness, health and human needs.* Washington, DC: National Academy Press.

Interagency Council on the Homeless. (1991). *The 1990 annual report.* Washington, DC: Author.

Interagency Council on the Homeless. (1994). *Priority: Home!* Washington, DC: Author.

Jacobs, F. H. (1994). Defining a social problem: the case of family homelessness. *American Behavioral Scientist,* 37 (3), 396-403.

Johnson, A. K., & Kreuger, L.W. (1989). Toward a better understanding of homeless women. *Social Work,* 34, 537-540.

Judd, C. M., & Kenny, D. A. (1981). *Estimating the effects of social interventions.* Cambridge, MA: Cambridge University Press.

The Kaiser Commission on the Future of Medicaid (1995). *Medicaid in transition.* Washington, DC: The Henry J. Kaiser Family Foundation.

Kaplan, T. (1995). *Health care coverage effects of the Wisconsin welfare reform proposal.* Madison, WI: Institute for Research on Poverty.

Kaufman, T. L. (1997). Out of reach: rental housing at what cost? *Journal of Housing and Community Development*, 54 (6), 25-30.

Kennedy, R. (1998, March 4). Availability of rent aid is reduced. *The New York Times,* pp. B1, B6.

Kilborn, P. T. (1998, March 22). Looking back at Jackson Hole. *The New York Times,* p. 16.

Kleinman, J. C., Gold, M., & Makuc, D. (1981). Use of ambulatory medical care by the poor: Another look at equity. *Medical Care,* 19 (10), 1011-1029.

Knickman, J. R., Weitzman, B. C., Shinn M., & Marcus, E. H. (1989). *A study of homeless families in New York City: Characteristics and comparisons with other public assistance families* (Final Report: Volume 2). New York: New York University, Robert F. Wagner Graduate School of Public Service, Health Research Program.

Kronick, R., Dreyfus, T. (1998). The challenge of risk adjustment for people with disabilities: Health-based payment for Medicaid health plans. *News and Strategies for Managed Medicare & Medicaid,* 4 (8), 4-6.

Kuder, J. M., & Levitz, G. S. (1989). Visits to the physician: An evaluation of the usual-source effect. In G. H. DeFriese, III, T. C. Ricketts, & J. S. Stein (Eds.), *Methodological advances in health services research,* (pp. 193-209). Ann Arbor, MI: Health Administration Press.

Lewin-Epstein, N. (1991). Determinants of regular source of health care in Black, Mexican, Puerto Rican, and Non-Hispanic white populations. *Medical Care*, 29 (6), 543-557.

Li, G. (1985). Robust Regression. In D. C. Hoaglin, F. Mosteller, & J. Tukey (Eds.), *Exploring Data Tables, Trends, Trends and Shapes* (pp. 281-340). New York: John Wiley & Sons.

Light, D. W. (1994). Managed care: False and real solutions. *The Lancet*, 344 (October 29), 1197-1199.

Link, B. G., Susser, E., Stueve, A., Phelan, J., Moore, R. E., & Struening, E. (1994). Lifetime and fiveyear prevalence of homelessness in the United States. *American Journal of Public Health*, 84 (12), 1907-1912.

Lipson, J. (1997). Medicaid managed care and community providers: New partnerships. *Health Affairs*, 16 (4), 91-107.

Litman, T. J. (1974). The family as a basic unit in health and medical care: A social behavioral overview. *Social Science Medicine*, 8, 495-519.

Litman, T. J., & Venters, M. (1979). Research on health care and the family: A methodological overview. *Social Science Medicine*, 13a, 379-385.

Markides, K. S., Levin, J. S., & Ray, L. A. (1985). Determinants of physician utilization among Mexican-Americans. *Medical Care*, 23 (3), 236-246.

Marquis, M. S. & Long, S. H. (1996). Reconsidering the effect of Medicaid on health services use. *Health Services Research*, 30 (6), 791-807.

Mayor's Office on Homelessness and SRO Housing for the City of New York. (1992). *Fact Sheet: Homelessness in New York City*. New York: City of New York.

Mayor's Advisory Council on Child Health. (1993). *Medicaid managed care in New York City: How will children fare?* New York: Child Health Action Management Plan.

McDonald, J. & Moffitt, R. (1980). The use of tobit analysis. *Review of Economics and Statistics*, 62, 318-321.

McKinlay, J. B. (1975). The health-seeking behavior of the poor. In J. Kosa, & I. K. Zola (Eds.), *Poverty and health: A sociological analysis* (pp. 224-273). Cambridge, MA: Harvard University Press.

Mead, L. M. (1992). *The New Politics of Poverty*. New York: Basic Books.

Mechanic, D. (1978). *Medical Sociology*. New York: The Free Press.

Mechanic, D. (1979). Correlates of physician utilization: Why do major multivariate studies of physician utilization find trivial psychosocial and organizational effects? *Journal of Health and Social Behavior*, 20, 387-396.

Mechanic, D. (1989). Medical sociology: Some tensions among theory, method, and substance. *Journal of Health and Social Behavior*, 30, 147-160.

Mechanic, D., & Aiken, L. (1989). Chapter 9: Access to health care and use of medical care services. In H. E. Freeman, & S. Levine (Eds.), *Handbook of Medical Sociology* (4th ed., pp. 166-242), Englewood Cliffs, NJ: Prentice Hall.

Milburn, N., & D'Ercole, A. (1991). Homeless women: Moving toward a comprehensive model. *American Psychologist*, 46 (11), 1161-1169.

Miller, D. S., & Lin, E. H. B. (1988). Children in sheltered homeless families: Reported health status and use of health services. *Pediatrics*, 81(5), 668-673.

Moffitt, R., & Wolfe, B. (1992). The effect of the Medicaid program on welfare participation and labor supply. *The Review of Economics and Statistics*, 74, 615-626.

Mohr, L. B. (1988). *Impact analysis for program evaluation*. Chicago: The Dorsey Press.

Molnar, J. M., Rath, W. R., & Klein. (1990). Constantly compromised: The impact of homelessness on children. *Journal of Social Issues*, 46 (4), 109-124.

Montgomery, J., & Fewer, W. (1988). *Family systems and beyond*. New York: Human Sciences Press, Inc.

Moore, P., & Hepworth, J. T. (1994). Use of perinatal and infant health services by MexicanAmerican Medicaid enrollees. *JAMA*, 272 (July 27), 297-304.

Muller, C. (1986). Review of twenty years of research on medical care utilization. *Health Services Research*, 21 (2), 129-144.

Nacmias, D., & Nachmias, C. (1981). *Research methods in the social sciences*. New York: St. Martin's Press.

National Center for Health Statistics. (1992). *National Ambulatory Medical Care Survey 1989*, (series 13, No. 110) Washington, DC: US Government Printing Office.

National Center for Health Statistics. (1994). *National Health Interview Survey 1992*, Washington, DC: US Government Printing Office.

Nattell, T., Pulver, W. (1996, October). *HIV prevalence among pregnant homeless women served by a mobile prenatal care clinic in New York City*. Paper presented at the meeting of the American Public Health Association, New York, NY.

Newacheck, P. W., & Butler, L. H. (1983). Patterns of physician use among lowincome, chronically ill persons. *Medical Care*, 21 (10), 981-989.

Newacheck, P.W., & Halfron, N. H. (1986). Access to ambulatory care services for economically disadvantaged children. *Pediatrics*, 87 (5), 813-818.

New York State Department of Health. (1998, March). HIV/AIDS quarterly updates. (www:Health.state.ny.us/nysdoh/aids/mar98/table2b.htm). Albany, NY: Author.

Nyamathi, A., Bennett, C., Leake, B., Lewis, C. & Flaskerud, J. (1993). AIDS-related knowledge, perceptions, and behaviors among impoverished minority women. *American Journal of Public Health*, 83 (1), 65-71.

Office of AIDS Surveillance. (1994). *AIDS surveillance update, 4th Quarter 1993*. New York: City of New York, Department of Health.

Office of Medicaid Managed Care. (1996, June). *Medicaid model contract for fully capitated managed care providers under the Partnership Plan*. New York: Medical Assistance Program, City of New York.

Office of Mental Health. (1988). Programs for homeless children and families. *Homelessness performance report*, Albany, NY: Department of Social Services, State of New York.

Office of Vital Statistics. (1992). *Summary of vital statistics 1989*. New York: Department of Health.

Orr, S. T., Charney, E., Straus, J., & Bloom, B. (1991). Emergency room use by low income children with a regular source of health care. *Medical Care*, 29 (3), 283-286.

Padgett, D., Struening, E., & Andrews, H. (1990). Factors affecting the use of medical, mental health, alcohol, and drug treatment services by homeless adults. *Medical Care*, 28 (9), 805-821.

Pavetti, L. A. (1996, May 23). *Time on welfare and welfare dependency*. (Testimony presented to the House of Representatives Committee on Ways and Means Subcommittee on Human Resources, 104th Congress). Washington, DC: Urban Institute.

Pear, R. (1997, December 29). Clinton ordering effort to sign up Medicaid children. *The New York Times*, pp. 1, 15.

Pomeroy, R. (1969). *Studies in the use of health services by families on welfare*. New York: City University of New York, The Center for the Study of Urban Problems.

Poland, B. D., Taylor, M. S., & Hayes, M. V. (1990). The ecology of health services utilization in Grenada, West Indies. *Social Science Medicine*, 30 (1), 13-24.

Pratt, L. (1976). *Family structure and effective health behavior: The energized family*. Boston: Houghton Mifflin Co.

Quint, J., Bos, J., & Polit, D. (1997). *New Chance: Final Report on a Comprehensive Program for Young Mothers in Poverty and Their Children.* New York: Manpower Demonstration Research Corporation.

Rafferty, Y., & Shinn, M. (1991). The Impact of homelessness on children. *American Psychologist,* 46 (11), 1170-1179.

Reed, W. L. (1990). Racism and health: The case of Black infant mortality, in P. Conrad and R. Kern (Eds.), *The Sociology of Health and Illness* (3rd ed., pp. 34-44). New York: St. Martin's Press.

Robertson, M. J. (1991). Homeless women with children: The role of alcohol and other drug abuse. *American Psychologist,* 46 (11), 1198-1204.

Rosenbaum, S., Hughes, D. C., & Johnson, K. (1988). Maternal and child health services for medically indigent children and pregnant women. *Medical Care,* 26 (4), 315-331.

Rosenthal, E. (1996, May 24). Mayor's stalled plans leave public hospitals in trauma. *The New York Times,* p. 1.

Rossi, P. H. (1994). Troubling Families: Family homelessness in America. *American Behavioral Scientist,* 37, 342-395.

Rowland, D., & Hanson, K. (1996). Medicaid: Moving to managed care. *Health Affairs,* 15 (3), 150-167.

Rowland, D., & Salganicoff, A. (1994). Commentary: Lessons from Medicaid: Improving access to office-based physicians care for the lowincome population. *American Journal of Public Health,* 84 (4), 550-552.

Saver, B. G., & Peterfreund, N. (1993). Insurance, income, and access to ambulatory care in King County, Washington. *American Journal of Public Health,* 83 (11), 1583-1588.

Shinn, M., Knickman, J. R., Ward, D., Petrovic, N. L., & Muth, B. J. (1990). Alternative models for sheltering homeless families. *Journal of Social Issues,* 46 (4), 175-190.

Shinn, M., Knickman, J. R., Weitzman, B.C. (1991). Social relationships and vulnerability to becoming homeless among families. *American Psychologist,* 46, 1190-1187.

Shinn, M., & Weitzman, B. C. (1994). You can't eliminate homelessness without housing. *American Behavioral Scientist,* 37 (3), 435-442.

Shinn, M., & Weitzman, B. C. (1996). Homeless families are different. In J. Baumohl (Ed.), *Homelessness in America: A reference book* (pp. 109-122). New York: Oryx Press.

Shinn M., Weitzman B. C., Stojanovic, D., Knickman J.R., Jimenez L., Duchon L., James S., Krantz D. (1998). Predictors of homelessness from shelter request to housing stability among families in New York City. *American Journal of Public Health*, 88 (12), in press.

Short, P. F., Cantor, J. C., & Monheit, A. C. (1988). The dynamics of Medicaid enrollment. *Inquiry*, 25 (Winter), 504-516.

Showstack, J., Lurie, N., Leatherman, S., Fisher, E., & Inui, T. (1996). Health of the public: Private sector challenge. *JAMA*, 276 (October 2), 1071-1074.

Singer, M. (1994). AIDS and the health crisis of the U.S. urban poor: The perspective of critical medical anthropology. *Social Science Medicine*, 39 (7), 931-947.

Smith, E. M., & North, C. S. (1994). Not all homeless women are alike: Effects of motherhood and the presence of children. *Community Mental Health Journal*, 30 (6), 601-610.

Sosin, M., Piliavin, I., & Westerfelt, H. (1990). Toward a longitudinal analysis of homelessness. *Journal of Social Issues*, 46 (4), 157-174.

Sparer, M. S. (1996). Medicaid managed care and the health reform debate: lessons from New York and California. *Journal of Health Politics, Policy, and Law*, 21 (3), 433-459.

The Stanford Center for the Study of Families, Children & Youth. (1991). *The nine studies of homeless families, children and youth*. Stanford, CA: Author.

State of New York. (1995). *The Partnership Plan*. Presented to the Secretary of Health and Human Services and the Administration of the Health Care Financing Administration, Albany, NY: Author.

Stokols, D., & Shumaker, S. A. (1982). The psychological context of residential mobility and wellbeing. *Journal of Social Issues*, 38 (3), 149-171.

Szapiro, N. (1988). Children, poverty, and hospital care in New York City. In M. I. Krasner (Ed.), *Poverty and health in New York City* (pp. 81-101). New York: United Hospital Fund.

Tanner, J. L., Cocherham, W. C., & Spaeth, J. L. (1983). Predicting physician utilization. *Medical Care*, 21 (3), 360-369.

Thrasher, S. P., & Mowbray, C. T. (1995). A strengths perspective: An ethnographic study of homeless women with children. *Health & Social Work*, 20 (5), 93-101.

Tobias, C. (1997). *Managed care for special populations: Developing responsive provider networks*. Princeton, NJ: Center for Health Care Strategies, Inc.

Toro, P. A., Trickett, E. J., Wall, D. D., & Salem, D. A. (1991). Homelessness in the United States: An ecological perspective. *American Psychologist*, 46 (11), 1208-1218.

Torrens, P. R. (1988). Historical Evolution and Overview of Health Services in the United States. In S. J. Williams & P. R. Torrens (Eds.), *Introduction to Health Services* (pp. 3-31). New York: John Wiley & Sons.

Toy, V. S. (1998, April 15). Tough workfare rules used as way to cut welfare rolls. *The New York Times*, pp. 1, B4.

United Hospital Fund (1992). *Health Care Annual*. New York: Author.

United Hospital Fund (1994). *New York City Community Health Atlas*. New York: Author.

U.S. Census Public Use Microdata Files for New York City borough totals, 1990, as cited in Moss, M., Townsend A., Tobier, E. (1997, December). *Immigration is transforming New York City*. New York: New York University, Robert F. Wagner Graduate School of Public Service, Taub Urban Research Center.

Urban Institute. (1997, November). *Welfare recipients and work: What can be expected?* (Issue No. 27, Update). Washington, DC: Author.

Urban Institute. (1998). *Health insurance for US children: Ten basic questions answered* (website:www.urban.org/news/factsheets/healthFS.html). Washington, DC: Author.

Vedlitz, A., & Alston, J. (1983). Welfare terminations and benefit reductions: What program recipients can tell policy planners. In R. Goldstein & S. Sachs (Eds.), *Applied Poverty Research* (pp. 138-147). Totowa, NJ: Rowman & Allanheld.

Wan, T. T. H., & Soifer, S. J. (1974). Determinants of physician utilization: A causal analysis. *Journal of Health & Social Behavior*, 15 (June), 100-107.

Ware, J. E., Bayliss, M. S., Rogers, W. H., Kosinski, M., & Tarlov, A. R. (1996). Differences in 4-year health outcomes for elderly and poor, chronically ill patients treated in HMO and fee-for-service systems. *JAMA*, 276 (October 2), 1039-1047.

Watson, J. M., & Kemper, K. J. (1995). Maternal factors and children's health care use. *Social Science Medicine*, 40 (5), 623-628.

Weeks, M. R., Schensul, J. J., Williams, S. S., Singer M., & Grier, M. (1995). AIDS prevention for African-American and Latina women: Building culturally and gender-appropriate intervention. *AIDS Education & Prevention*, 7 (3), 251-264.

Weil, A. (1997, October). *The new children's health insurance program: Should states expand Medicaid?* (No. A-13 in series, New federalism: Issues and options for states). Washington, DC: Urban Institute.

Weiner, J. P., Starfield, B. H., Powe, N. R., Stuart, M. E., & Steinwachs, D. M. (1996). Ambulatory care practice variation within a Medicaid program. *Health Services Research*, 30 (6), 751-769.

Weitzman, B. C. (1989). Pregnancy and childbirth: Risk factors for homelessness? *Family Planning Perspectives*, 21 (4), 175-178.

Weitzman, B. C., Knickman, J. R., & Shinn, M. (1990). Pathways to homelessness among New York City families. *Journal of Social Issues*, 46 (4), 125-140.

Weitzman, B. C., Knickman, J. R., & Shinn, M. (1992). Predictors of shelter use among lowincome families: Psychiatric history, substance abuse, and victimization. *American Journal of Public Health*, 82 (11), 1547-1550.

Wells, K. B., Golding, J. M., Hough, R. L., Burnam, A., & Karno, M. (1988). Factors affecting the probability of use of general and medical health and social/community services for Mexican Americans and non-Hispanic whites. *Medical Care*, 26 (5), 441-452.

Wiecha, J. L., Dwyer, J. T., & DunnStrohecker, M. (1991). Nutrition and health services needs among the homeless. *Public Health Reports*, 106 (4), 364-373.

Wilson, W. J. & Neckerman, K. M. (1986). Poverty and family structure: The widening gap between evidence and public policy issues. In S.H. Danziger and D. H. Weinberg (Eds.), *Fighting Poverty* (pp. 232-259). Cambridge, MA: Harvard University Press.

Winkleby, M. A., & Boyce, W. T. (1994). Healthrelated risk factors of homeless families and single adults. *Journal of Community Health*, 19 (February), 7-23.

Winterbottom, C., Liska, D., Obermaier, K. (1995). *State-level databook on health care access and financing*, (2nd ed.), Washington, DC: The Urban Institute.

Wiseman, M. (1996). State strategies for welfare reform: The Wisconsin story. *Journal of Policy Analysis and Management*, 15 (4), 515-545.

Wolfe, B. L. (1980). Children's utilization of medical care. *Medical Care*, 18 (12), 1196-1207.

Wolfe, S., & Badgley, R. (1972). Patients and their families. *Milbank Memorial Fund* Quarterly, 50, Part II (2), 69-89.

Wolinsky, F. D. (1978). Assessing the effects of predisposing, enabling and illness-morbidity characteristics on health service utilization. *Journal of Health and Social Behavior*, 19, 384-396.

Wolinsky, F. D. (1981). The problems for academic and entrepreneurial research in the use of health services. *The Sociological Quarterly*, 22, 207-223.

Wolinsky, F. D. (1982). Assessing the effects of the physical, psychological, and social dimensions of health on the use of health services. *The Sociological Quarterly*, 23, 191-206.

Wolinsky, F. D. (1988). *The sociology of health: Principles, practitioners, and issues* (2nd ed.). Belmont, CA: Wadsworth Publishing Co.

Women's City Club of New York. (1992). *Beyond Facilities and Good Intentions*, New York: The Coalition for the Homeless.

Wood, D., Halfron, N., Sherbourne, C., & Grabowsky, M. (1994). Access to infant immunizations for poor inner-city families: What is the impact of managed care? *Journal of Health Care for the Poor and Underserved*, 5 (2), 112-123.

Wood, D., & Valdez, R. B. (1991). Barriers to medical care for homeless families compared with housed poor families. *American Journal of Diseases of Children*, 145 (10), 1109-1115.

Wood, D., Valdez, R. B., Hayashi, T., & Shen, A. (1990). Homeless and housed families in Los Angeles: A study comparing demographic, economic, and family function characteristics. *American Journal of Public Health*, 80, 1049-1052.

Wright, J. D., & Weber, E. (1988). Determinants of benefit-program participation among the urban homeless. *Evaluation Review*, 12 (4), 376-395.

Zedlewski, S., Clark, S., Meier, E., & Watson, K. (1996). *Potential effects of congressional welfare reform legislation family incomes*. Washington, DC: The Urban Institute.

Zlotnick, C., Kronstadt, D., & Klee, L. (1996, October). *Foster care children, their parents and the cycle of homelessness*. Paper presented at the meeting of the American Public Health Association, New York, NY.

Zuckerman, B. & Beardslee, W. R. (1987). Maternal depression: A concern for pediatricians. *Pediatrics*, 79, 110.

For Product Safety Concerns and Information please contact our EU representative GPSR@taylorandfrancis.com
Taylor & Francis Verlag GmbH, Kaufingerstraße 24, 80331 München, Germany

www.ingramcontent.com/pod-product-compliance
Lightning Source LLC
LaVergne TN
LVHW021109300926
849160LV00009B/662

* 9 7 8 1 1 3 8 9 6 9 5 3 7 *